Christian F. Poets
Axel Franz
Petra Koehne

**Controversies around treatment
of the open duct**

Christian F. Poets
Axel Franz
Petra Koehne

Controversies around treatment of the open duct

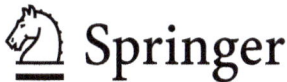
Springer

Christian F. Poets
Universitätsklinikum Tübingen
Neonatologie
Calwerstr. 7
72076 Tübingen

Petra Koehne
Charité Universitätsmedizin Berlin
Klinik für Neonatologie
Augustenburger Platz 1
13353 Berlin

Axel Franz
Universitätsklinikum Tübingen
Neonatologie
Calwerstr. 7
72076 Tübingen

ISBN-13   978-3-642-20622-1 Springer-Verlag Berlin Heidelberg New York

Bibliographic information Deutsche Bibliothek
The Deutsche Bibliothek lists this publication in Deutsche Nationalbibliographie;
detailed bibliographic data is available in the internet at <http://dnb.ddb.de>.

SpringerMedizin
Springer-Verlag GmbH
ein Unternehmen von Springer Science+Business
springer.de

© Springer-Verlag Berlin Heidelberg 2011

Planning: Diana Kraplow
Project management: Diana Kraplow
Cover design: deblik Berlin
Typesetting and reproduction of the figures:
Fotosatz-Service Köhler GmbH – Reinhold Schöberl, Würzburg

18/5141 – 5 4 3 2 1 0   SPIN 80061200

Preface

The patent ductus arteriosus continues to pose a considerable challenge to clinicians and scientists alike. Why does it close spontaneously in most infants but remain open in others? How best can we select those infants who are most likely to benefit from treatment, i.e. are there echocardiographic criteria that would help in defining a more selective treatment approach? Would it be better to take an aggressive approach and prescribe prophylactic treatment to all extremely immature infants and if so, what is the best way to define such a subgroup? Or should we rather be more restrictive in applying the current treatment indications and adopt a "wait and see" policy in most, if not all, premature infants? Finally, are there data to suggest that one of the treatment approaches that are available to close the patent ductus arteriosus is superior to the other?

These and other pressing questions were addressed during a meeting on the treatment of the patent ductus arteriosus, convened on September 30 to October 1, 2010, in Stuttgart, Germany. Presentations given during this meeting have been summarized by the authors for this book; they are supplemented by a report on the discussions that followed each lecture. This endeavour was made possible by the generous support of Orphan Europe; however, the contents of this book do not necessarily reflect the views of the company.

We hope that readers find the data presented here helpful in arriving at appropriate decisions when faced with the dilemma of how to deal with the patent ductus arteriosus best in their patients. Our sincere thanks to all the authors for their contributions – without their efforts this book would not have been possible.

Tübingen and Berlin, May 2011
Christian F. Poets, MD, Axel Franz, MD, and Petra Koehne, MD

Table of Contents

Evaluation of the Open Duct Using Systolic Time Intervals and Doppler Sonography of Peripheral Arteries

Competitive Inhibition of Bilirubin-Albumin Binding by Ibuprofen

List of Contributors

Sofia Aliaga, MD, MPH
School of Medicine
Division of Neonatal-Perinatal
Medicine
The University of North Carolina
at Chapel Hill
Chapel Hill, NC

Bernd Beedgen, MD
Klinik Kinderheilkunde IV
(Schwerpunkt Neonatologie),
Zentrum für Kinder-
und Jugendmedizin,
Universitätsklinikum Heidelberg
Im Neuenheimer Feld 430
69120 Heidelberg, Germany
bernd.beedgen@med.
uni-heidelberg.de

Regina Bökenkamp, MD
Abteilung Kinderheilkunde III
Pädiatrische Kardiologie
und Pädiatrische Intensivmedizin
Medizinische Hochschule Hannover
Carl-Neuberg-Straße 1
30625 Hannover

Luc Desfrère, MD
Service de Néonatologie
Hôpital Louis Mourier, AP HP
Colombes
Université Paris 7
Faculté de Médecine Denis Diderot
Paris
France

Nick Evans DM, MRCPCH
Department of Newborn Care
Royal Prince Alfred Hospital
Missenden Rd, Camperdown,
Sydney, New South Wales 2111
Australia
nevans@med.usyd.edu.au

Axel Franz, MD
Universitätsklinikum Tübingen
Neonatologie
Calwerstr. 7
72076 Tübingen

Pricilla Herrmann, MA
Center for Pediatric Clinical Studies
Frondsbergstraße 23
72076 Tübingen

Petra Koehne, MD
Charité Universitätsmedizin Berlin
Klinik für Neonatologie
Augustenburger Platz 1
13353 Berlin
petra.koehne@charite.de

Matthew M. Laughon, MD, MPH
School of Medicine
Division of Neonatal-Perinatal
Medicine
The University of North Carolina
at Chapel Hill
Chapel Hill, NC
matt_laughon@med.unc.edu

Eva Robel-Tillig, MD
Klinikum St. Georg
Fachbereich Neonatologie/
Pädiatrische Intensivmedizin
Delitzscher Str. 141
04129 Leipzig

Bart Van Overmeire, MD, PhD
Head of Neonatal Intensive Care
Unit
Professor of Paediatrics
Erasmus Hospital – ULB, Université
Libre de Bruxelles
Brussels
Belgium

Ductal Closure After Birth – Morphological Aspects and New Insights

R. Bökenkamp

1

Introduction

Although the uniqueness of the ductus arteriosus (DA) as a foetal structure was already described in antique medicine by Galen [1] research into mechanisms underlying the neonatal closing process is ongoing. The motivation to study ductal closure after birth is diverse among the different specialities. Basic researchers are interested in the physiological remodelling process that starts early in foetal life [2] because of its similarities with other vascular remodelling processes such as vascular ageing and atherosclerosis. Clinicians wish to prevent morbidity in premature infants associated with delayed postnatal ductal closure and also in neonates with duct-dependent cardiac defects who can be rescued by a patent DA.

Developmental Background

Before the left 6th pharyngeal arch artery undergoes the DA-specific differentiation programme, the vascular system of the embryo develops from an endothelial plexus derived from the splanchnic mesoderm. After folding of the embryo the endothelial plexus in the heart region becomes incorporated within the myocardium [3]. The omphalomesenteric vessels enter the heart at the venous pole, while the arterial pole becomes connected to the dorsal aortae by the symmetric pharyngeal arches. Arteries develop after endothelial cells (EC) have recruited cells that differentiate into smooth muscle cells (SMC). Patterning of the pharyngeal arches [4] is influenced by neural crest cells, second heart field derived cells and by the neuronal system surrounding the arches [5, 6]. Differences in matrix production and growth are responsible for the development of the SMC phenotype [5].

Ductal Maturation

The early second trimester human foetus has a muscular DA with a single or locally duplicated internal elastic lamina and a very thin intima. With advancing development the internal elastic lamina becomes fragmented and intimal cushions increase in size [2]. After full gestation the intimal cushions are large enough to seal the ductal lumen probably in concert with a platelet thrombus

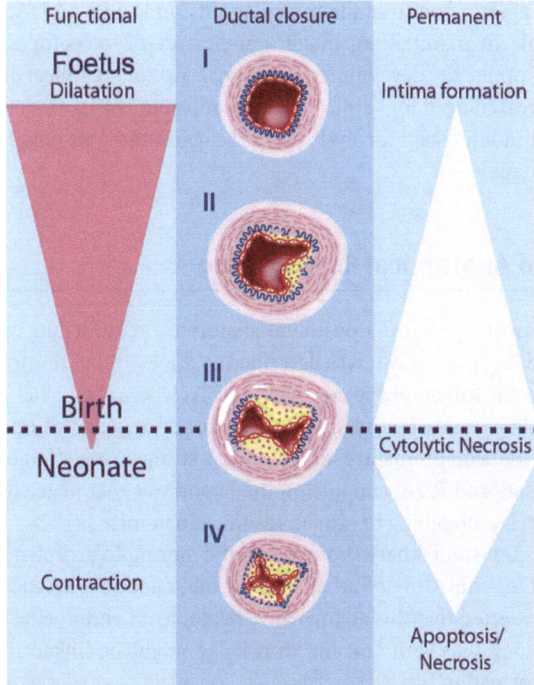

Fig. 1.1. Schematic overview of the histological features related to maturation and anatomical closure of the human ductus arteriosus. The histological maturity stages are derived from Gittenberger et al. [2]. At the end of the first trimester of pregnancy the DA is in the immature stage I. This stage is characterized by the lack of intimal thickening. The endothelial cells (ECs) are firmly attached to the internal elastic lamina (IEL). During the second trimester the DA enters the intermediate stage II. The EC are lifted form the fragmenting IEL. Intimal thickening develops. The mature DA in stage III has abundant intimal cushions and a fragmented IEL. Apoptosis and cytolytic necrosis develop in the inner media. After mature birth it is most likely that the normal DA enters stage IV and shows complete closure. The ductus finally degenerates into a fibrous remnant through apoptosis and necrosis

[7] when the vessel contracts under the influence of oxygen and prostaglandin withdrawal. In the weeks after birth the functionally closed DA degenerates as a consequence of cytolytic necrosis and apoptosis into the ligamentum arteriosum [8]. ▪ Figure 1.1 gives a schematic overview over the histologic features. Experimental data [9–11] from prostaglandin-receptor EP4-disrupt-

ed mice suggest a dual role for prostglandins on the foetal DA. Besides its primary role in maintaining ductal patency, PGE2-receptor activation is shown to promote the development of intimal cushions. Clinical data describing the increased need for surgical ligation of patent DA in premature infants born after indomethacin tocolysis [12, 13] suggest that this might also be the case in humans.

Postnatal Anatomical Remodelling

The mechanisms governing postnatal anatomical remodelling are not fully understood. Very recently it was described in mice [7] that thrombocytes are recruited to the lumen of the constricting DA, where they block blood flow and probably promote remodelling to achieve permanent closure.

Clinical data on premature infants show a strong association between low platelet counts and PDA, supporting the hypothesis that platelets play a key role in ductal remodelling in humans as they do in mice [7].

Histological studies have shown a specific morphological characteristic in persistent DA, consisting of an additional subendothelial elastic membrane [14]. It is expected that this abnormality relates to an endothelial differentiation deficiency that with current knowledge might be linked to disturbed thrombus formation [8].

PDA in Premature Infants – Morphologic Aspects

The DA of a premature infant will generally not have passed through all stages of maturation. However, gestational age alone is not sufficient to predict whether the DA of a preterm infant is likely to close at the time of birth [15]. Histological studies documented no strict relation between gestational age or birthweight and the maturational stage of the DA shown in ◘ Fig. 1.1. This explains that early spontaneous closure of the DA is possible even in a young premature infant.

Signalling Related to Ductal Closure

For decades, the constrictive effect of oxygen on the DA in the neonate [16] as well as the relaxing effect of prostaglandins [17] have been shown. Studies in various animal species and in-vitro models revealed additional mediators for DA regulation and remodelling. Species differences in the degree, timing, and type of reaction to various stimuli have been documented. ◘ Figure 1.2 shows a compilation of these experimental in-vitro- and in-vivo data reviewed in Bokenkamp et al. [18] in order to illustrate parallel actions and potential interactions of the various signalling pathways.

Genetic and Environmental Risk Factors for PDA in Premature Infants

Absence of antenatal glucocorticoid treatment [19] and immaturity are established environmental risk factors for PDA in premature infants. Recently, genetic contributions to PDA in this patient population were studied by several groups [20–22]. The finding that PDA is significantly more prevalent than expected in both individuals of prematurely born twin pairs supports the role of a genetic factor [22]. Studies on PDA in preterm infants revealed polymorphisms in the *TFAP2B* gene [20, 21], a gene that is mutated in Char syndrome, a condition comprising PDA, facial dysmorphism and abnormal fifth digits. Furthermore, sequence polymorphisms in various additional genes were found in premature infants with PDA. The recent finding of decreased RNA expression of three calcium and potassium channel-genes in humans carrying a *TFAP2B* DNA polymorphism [21], suggests that transcriptional regulation of these ion channels may play a role in postnatal DA closure.

Prevention of DA Closure in Neonates with CHD

The discovery that prostaglandins are responsible for ductal patency during foetal life [17] is the basis of the present pharmacological approach to the DA. In neonates with duct-dependent congenital heart defects systemic application of synthetic prostaglandins ensures ductal patency until the cardiac lesion can be treated surgically or by catheter-intervention. As PGE treatment has a

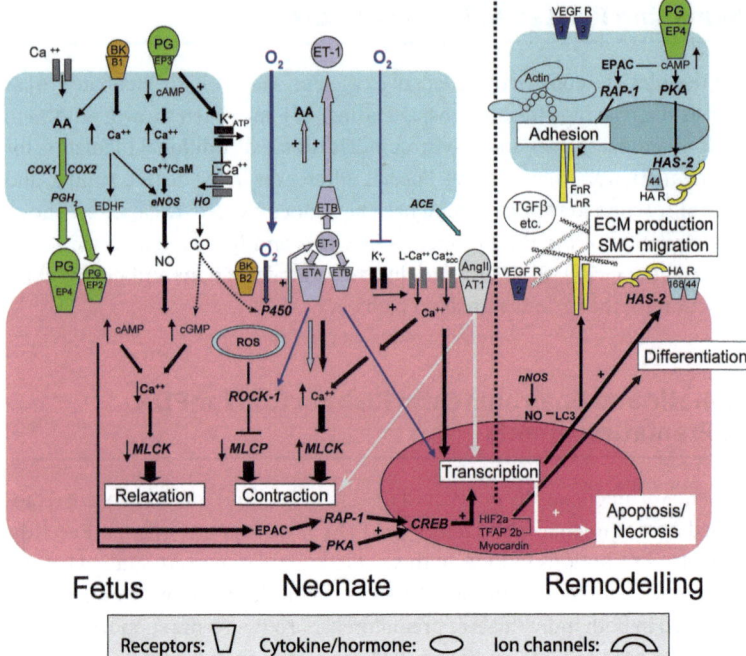

wide range of systemic [23] and local side-effects [24], one should be prepared to modify treatment regimens according to the changing clinical practice. For example, the antenatal diagnosis of heart defects has the advantage that neonates need a lower starting dose of PGE immediately after birth, because their DA has not closed yet. Lower PGE doses reduce the dose-dependent risk of developing apnoea, thereby offering more safety for the infant during transport [25]. New catheter-based and hybrid therapies for the treatment of certain cardiac malformations [26, 27] place stents in the DA to prevent closure in the longer term. For the safety of these interventions it is desirable to control the diameter of the ductus arteriosus accurately and keep its wall structure intact.

◀ ◻ **Fig. 1.2.** Diagram of the signalling pathways involved in ductal remodelling and post-natal closure. Endothelial cells (ECs) are depicted in light blue. Vascular smooth muscle cells (VSMCs) are indicated by the large pink rectangle. For the sake of clarity, not all downstream signalling steps are included. On the left side, the dominant signalling pathways in the foetus are shown. The middle section illustrates the changes related to the increase of oxygen saturation at birth. The section to the right of the vertical dotted line focuses on anatomical remodelling. Remodelling proceeds through a sequence of events including the differentiation of VSMCs and ECs, extracellular matrix production, VSMC migration, and finally apoptosis and necrosis.

Abbreviations: *AA* arachidonic acid, *ACE* angiotensin-converting enzyme, *Ang II* angiotensin II with AT1 receptor, *BK* bradykinin with receptors B1 and B2, Ca^{++} calcium ion and channels: Ca_{SOC} store operated, *L-Ca* voltage-dependent; *CaM* calmodulin, *cAMP* cyclic adenosine monophosphate, *cGMP* cyclic guanosine monophosphate, *CO* carbon monoxide, *COX* cycloxygenase isoforms 1 and 2, *CREB* cAMP response element-binding protein, *ECM* extracellular matrix, *EDHF* endothelium hyperpolarising factor, *EPAC* exchange proteins activated by cAMP, *ET-1* endothelin-1 with ET-A and ET-B receptors, *HAS-2* hyaluronansynthase-2, *FnR* fibronectin receptor, *HA* hyaluronic acid receptors, *CD 44 and CD168* receptors for hyaluronic acid mediated motility, *HIF-2a* hypoxia-inducible factor 2 alpha, *HO* hemoxygenase, K^+ potassium ion and channels: K_{ATP} ATP-sensitive channel, *Kv* voltage-gated channel; *LC3* microtubule-associated protein, *LnR* laminin receptor, *MLCK* myosin light-chain kinase, *MLCP* myosin light chain phosphatase, *NO* nitric oxide, *NOS* nitric oxide synthase isoforms (endothelial) eNOS and (neuronal) nNOS, *PGH2* prostaglandin H2, *PG* prostaglandins in the predominantly PGE2 and PGI2 acting via prostaglandin receptors (EP 2,3,4), *PKA* protein kinase A, *RAP1* small RAS-like GTPase acting downstream of EPAC, *ROCK-1* Rho-associated, coiled-coil-containing protein kinase 1, *ROS* reactive oxygen species, *TFAP2b* transcription-factor-activating protein 2 beta, *SOC* store-operated channel, *VEGF* vascular endothelial growth factor

Conclusion

Ductal closure after birth is mediated by two processes: constriction and anatomical remodelling. In-utero constriction is counteracted mainly by prostaglandins and low oxygen partial pressure. Anatomical remodelling initiates in this intrauterine environment as a result of highly orchestrated molecular interactions. Better understanding of these molecular mechanisms will help to develop new treatment strategies. In the future, genotype data may also be used to predict success of pharmacologic treatment and influence therapeutic decisions.

1

References

1. Galenus C (2010) Opera Omnia IV. 243
2. Gittenberger-de Groot AC, van E, I, Moulaert AJ, Harinck E (1980) The ductus arteriosus in the preterm infant: histologic and clinical observations. J Pediatr 96: 88–93
3. DeRuiter MC, Poelmann RE, VanderPlas-de V, I, Mentink MM, Gittenberger-de Groot AC (1992) The development of the myocardium and endocardium in mouse embryos. Fusion of two heart tubes? Anat Embryol (Berl) 185: 461–473
4. Molin DG, DeRuiter MC, Wisse LJ, Azhar M, Doetschman T, Poelmann RE, Gittenberger-de Groot AC (2002) Altered apoptosis pattern during pharyngeal arch artery remodelling is associated with aortic arch malformations in Tgfbeta2 knock-out mice. Cardiovasc Res 56: 312–322
5. Bergwerff M, DeRuiter MC, Gittenberger-de Groot AC (1999) Comparative anatomy and ontogeny of the ductus arteriosus, a vascular outsider. Anat Embryol (Berl) 200: 559–571
6. Rochais F, Mesbah K, Kelly RG (2009) Signaling pathways controlling second heart field development. Circ Res 104: 933–942
7. Echtler K, Stark K, Lorenz M et al. (2010) Platelets contribute to postnatal occlusion of the ductus arteriosus. Nat Med 16: 75–82
8. Slomp J, Gittenberger-de Groot AC, Glukhova MA, Conny van MJ, Kockx MM, Schwartz SM, Koteliansky VE (1997) Differentiation, dedifferentiation, and apoptosis of smooth muscle cells during the development of the human ductus arteriosus. Arterioscler Thromb Vasc Biol 17: 1003–1009
9. Yokoyama U, Minamisawa S, Quan H et al. (2006) Chronic activation of the prostaglandin receptor EP4 promotes hyaluronan-mediated neointimal formation in the ductus arteriosus. J Clin Invest 116: 3026–3034
10. Segi E, Sugimoto Y, Yamasaki A et al. (1998) Patent ductus arteriosus and neonatal death in prostaglandin receptor EP4-deficient mice. Biochem Biophys Res Commun 246: 7–12
11. Nguyen M, Camenisch T, Snouwaert JN, Hicks E, Coffman TM, Anderson PA, Malouf NN, Koller BH (1997) The prostaglandin receptor EP4 triggers remodelling of the cardiovascular system at birth. Nature 390: 78–81
12. Hammerman C, Glaser J, Kaplan M, Schimmel MS, Ferber B, Eidelman AI (1998) Indomethacin tocolysis increases postnatal patent ductus arteriosus severity. Pediatrics 102: E56
13. Soraisham AS, Dalgleish S, Singhal N (2010) Antenatal indomethacin tocolysis is associated with an increased need for surgical ligation of patent ductus arteriosus in preterm infants. J Obstet Gynaecol Can 32: 435–442
14. Gittenberger-de Groot AC (1977) Persistent ductus arteriosus: most probably a primary congenital malformation. Br Heart J 39: 610–618
15. Gittenberger-de Groot AC, van E, I, Moulaert AJ, Harinck E (1980) The ductus arteriosus in the preterm infant: histologic and clinical observations. J Pediatr 96: 88–93
16. Heymann MA, Rudolph AM (1975) Control of the ductus arteriosus. Physiol Rev 55: 62–78

17. Coceani F, Olley PM, Bodach E (1975) Lamb ductus arteriosus: effect of prostaglandin synthesis inhibitors on the muscle tone and the response to prostaglandin E2. Prostaglandins 9: 299–308

18. Bokenkamp R, DeRuiter MC, van MC, Gittenberger-de Groot AC (2010) Insights into the pathogenesis and genetic background of patency of the ductus arteriosus. Neonatology 98: 6–17

19. Clyman RI, Mauray F, Roman C, Heymann MA, Ballard PL, Rudolph AM, Payne B (1981) Effects of antenatal glucocorticoid administration on ductus arteriosus of preterm lambs. Am J Physiol 241: H415–H420

20. Dagle JM, Lepp NT, Cooper ME et al. (2009) Determination of genetic predisposition to patent ductus arteriosus in preterm infants. Pediatrics 123: 1116–1123

21. Waleh N, Hodnick R, Jhaveri N et al. (2010) Patterns of gene expression in the ductus arteriosus are related to environmental and genetic risk factors for persistent ductus patency. Pediatr Res 68: 292–297

22. Bhandari V, Zhou G, Bizzarro MJ, Buhimschi C, Hussain N, Gruen JR, Zhang H (2009) Genetic contribution to patent ductus arteriosus in the premature newborn. Pediatrics 123: 669–673

23. Saxena A, Sharma M, Kothari SS, Juneja R, Reddy SC, Sharma R, Bhan A, Venugopal P (1998) Prostaglandin E1 in infants with congenital heart disease: Indian experience. Indian Pediatr 35: 1063–1069

24. Gittenberger-de Groot AC (1995) Histopathology of the ductus arteriosus after PGE1 treatment. Pediatr Cardiol 16: 101

25. Browning Carmo KA, Barr P, West M, Hopper NW, White JP, Badawi N (2007) Transporting newborn infants with suspected duct dependent congenital heart disease on low-dose prostaglandin E1 without routine mechanical ventilation. Arch Dis Child Fetal Neonatal Ed 92: F117–F119

26. Akinturk H, Michel-Behnke I, Valeske K, Mueller M, Thul J, Bauer J, Hagel KJ, Schranz D (2007) Hybrid transcatheter-surgical palliation: basis for univentricular or biventricular repair: the Giessen experience. Pediatr Cardiol 28: 79–87

27. Gewillig M, Boshoff DE, Dens J, Mertens L, Benson LN (2004) Stenting the neonatal arterial duct in duct-dependent pulmonary circulation: new techniques, better results. J Am Coll Cardiol 43: 107–112

Treatment Results After Ductal Closure in Extremely Low Gestational Age Infants

P. Koehne

Factors Determining Outcome of Very Low Birth Weight Infants

Preterm neonates weighing below 1500g at birth (i.e., very low birth weight (VLBW) infants) account for 1.5% of all live born infants in the European Union and have a survival rate above 85%, yet the handicap rate has not changed during the past decade [1]. These VLBW infants may suffer from severe motor dysfunction in 5% and complex developmental impairment in 15% to 20% of survivors [2–4]. In addition, 15% to 36% of these children have been reported to suffer major neurodevelopmental handicaps at school age [5, 6]. By age of 8 years, 25% have repeated at least one grade in school, and >50% are receiving special educational services [7, 8]. It is well known that impaired neurodevelopment is associated with several risk factors like degree of immaturity, male gender, poor social status and the presence of intraventricular hemorrhage (IVH), periventricular leukomalacia (PVL), necrotizing enterocolitis (NEC), bronchopulmonary dysplasia (BPD), sepsis or microcephalus [9].

Failure of spontaneous ductal closure occurs in 25% of VLBW infants and may promote organ damage due to a volume overload of the heart and lungs, but a cerebral and intestinal perfusion deficit [10, 11]. Because the combined goals of perinatal intensive care are to promote survival and to prevent handicap in this high-risk neonatal population, it is critical to examine factors that may affect developmental outcome and to evaluate the potential contribution of an open duct to impaired development.

Impact of Patent Ductus Arteriosus Intervention for Outcome

Despite a large number of studies that have been performed to evaluate the effects of interventions for patent ductus arteriosus (PDA), the possible impact of a PDA and its treatment on the long-term outcome of these infants is not clear. This is in part attributable to the fact that all studies have allowed subsequent rescue PDA treatment in the control groups and to scarce availability of follow-up data.

Prophylactic Cyclooxygenase Inhibitor Treatment

Although the majority of trials was set up for therapeutic PDA intervention the studies on prophylactic cyclooxygenase [12] inhibitor use involve the largest number of patients.

Prophylactic Intravenous Indomethacin

In a meta-analysis of 19 randomized trials, involving 2872 preterm infants ≤37 weeks gestational age with a birth weight ≤1750 g, the prophylactic use of indomethacin has been shown clear short-term benefits: a reduction in the incidence of severe IVH (IVH ≥3°, NNT 20), of later symptomatic PDA (NNT 4) and PDA ligation (NNT 20; ◘ Fig. 2.1) [13]. These results are not accompanied by any of the anticipated adverse outcomes that could have been expected given the vasoconstrictive nature of the drug – that is, important renal side effects, gastrointestinal perforation, and NEC [14]. However, the fact that prophylactic indomethacin fails to reduce short-term pulmonary morbidity, i.e. the incidence of BPD, challenges the notion that a persistently patent duct contributes to lung damage.

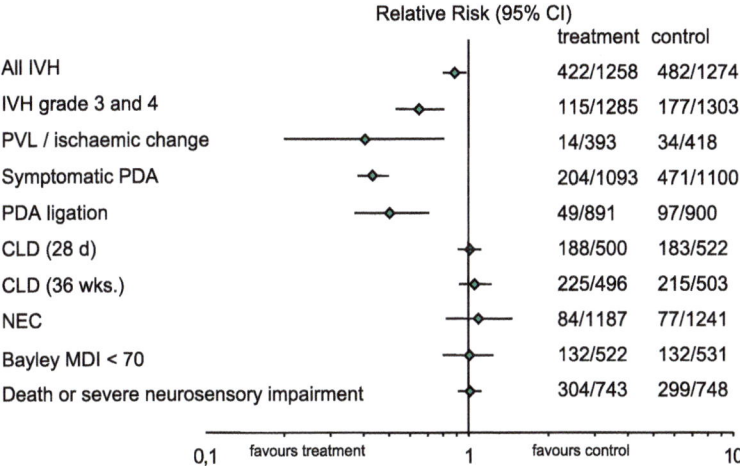

◘ **Fig. 2.1.** Meta-analysis of short and long-term outcomes observed in controlled trials with prophylactic intravenous indomethacin use. *IVH* intraventricular hemorrhage; *PVL* periventricular leukomalacia; *CLD* chronic lung disease; *NEC* necrotizing enterocolitis; *MDI* mental developmental index. (Adapted from Fowlie and Davis [13])

2

The timing of the prophylactic administration (<6 hours to <24 hours of life) as well as the dose regimen used (1 × 0,2 mg/kg indomethacin q 24 hours – 6 × 0,1 mg/kg on days 1.–6. of life) varied between individual trials. The two largest trials included in the analysis were the studies by the groups of Laura Ment (431 preterm infants) and Barbara Schmidt (TIPP, 1202 preterm infants) which accounted for 57% of the total study population, implicating that all conclusions drawn from this meta-analysis are heavily influenced by these two trials [15, 16].

Neurodevelopmental follow-up data are available from 3 studies up to the age of 18 months or two years in many children (Bandstra et al. – 199 preterm infants – Bayley MDI and PDI between 6 and 24 months; TIPP 2001 – 1202 preterm infants – Bayley MDI at 18 months) and to eight years in a smaller cohort (Ment et al. – 431 preterm infants – at 36 and 54 months and at school age) [16–20].

There is no evidence from the follow-up data to suggest either benefit or harm in longer term outcomes including the rates of survival without cognitive delay, cerebral palsy, blindness or deafness. A subgroup analysis of the TIPP trial based on birth weight (500–749 g and 750–999 g) revealed no significant differences in rates of composite adverse outcomes at 18 months in either subgroup (indomethacin 63% and 36% vs. control 61% and 35%). However, it has been suggested that the 18-months follow-up performed in the TIPP trial may have failed to detect subtle neurodevelopmental abnormalities that may become evident later in childhood. Bearing in mind that indomethacin alters cerebral blood flow to the developing brain and that the prophylactic treatment approach goes along with the unnecessary exposure of many infants to this drug, both subtle benefits – but also subtle harm from prophylactic administration is conceivable. The only long-term follow-up results exist from the randomized, prospective multicenter indomethacin IVH prevention trial conducted by the group of Laura Ment between 1989 and 1992 (◘ Table 2.1). Besides the primary outcome measure IVH at postnatal day 5, neurodevelopmental status at ages 3 to 8 years corrected age was a predefined secondary outcome. Assessments included the Peabody Picture Vocabulary Test and measures of intelligence at all ages. Of the 431 infants admitted to the original trial, 384 survived (192 of 209 infants receiving indomethacin, and 192 of 222 infants receiving saline placebo). There were no significant differences in the birth weights, proportions of male infants, maternal ages, or years of maternal education between the two groups. In addition, there were no

Table 2.1. Neurodevelopmental outcome of preterm infants in the Multicenter Indomethacin Intraventricular Hemorrhage Prevention Trial of Ment et al. [18–20]

	Indomethacin	Control	p
Survivors (384/431)	n=192 (92%)	n=192 (86%)	
Stanford-Binet IQ 36 months' CA (English-monolingual children)	89.6 + 18.92 n=126	85.0 + 20.79 n=122	n.s.
WPPSI Full scale 54 months' CA, IQ <70	11/119 (9%)	19/114 (17%)	0.04
PPVT-R, < 70	14/119 (12%)	28/114 (26%)	0.02
WISC-III Full scale, 8 years' CA without IVH	93.2 + 18 n=145	92.5 + 18 n=135	n.s.
PPVT-R, <70 without IVH	12/142 (8%)	24/131 (18%)	0.04

CA corrected age, *PPVT-R* Peabody Picture Vocabulary Test-Revised, *WPPSI* Wechsler Preschool and Primary Scale of Intelligence-Revised; *WISC-III* Wechsler Intelligence Scale for Children – Third Edition.

differences in the incidence of PVL, ventriculomegaly, and cerebral palsy between infants who received indomethacin and infants who received placebo. However, mean gestational age of the children randomized to receive indomethacin was significantly lower than that of the children randomized to receive placebo (27.7 vs 28.4 weeks). Categorical analysis of the data by Ment et al. revealed that indomethacin administered as prophylaxis against IVH in VLBW infants does not result in adverse cognitive or motor functioning at 3, 4 ½ and 8 years corrected age [18–20]. Some post-hoc analyses of the Ment cohort even suggested trends towards improved long-term outcome after prophylactic low-dose indomethacin, some of which became statistically significant with adjustment for certain baseline variables. Nevertheless, these post-hoc analyses cannot be considered confirmatory.

Because indomethacin has been shown to exhibit sex-specific effects on cerebrovascular reactivity [21], and since boys are more likely to have preterm birth and are at higher risk for numerous neonatal neurologic morbidities, it is interesting to look at the results from the cohort of Ment et al. analyzed ac-

2

■ **Table 2.2.** Peabody Picture Vocabulary Test-R scores of preterm infants in the Multicenter Indomethacin Intraventricular Hemorrhage Prevention Trial of Ment et al. [22]

	3 years	4.5 years	6 years	8 years
Female, n=196				
– Saline, n=103	88.5 ± 17.3	90.0 ± 21.7	92.0 ± 21.7	92.6 ± 22.3
– Indomethacin, n=93	83.5 ± 22.0	88.5 ± 22.0	93.2 ± 25.2	90.8 ± 24.8
Male*, n=235				
– Saline, n=119	77.8 ± 25.1	79.0 ± 29.8	86.8 ± 29.8	89.9 ± 30.0
– Indomethacin, n=116	87.4 ± 20.6	87.3 ± 19.9	96.6 ± 19.6	95.4 ± 23.4

Data are shown according to treatment, sex and corrected age. *$p < 0.05$ for male sex for all age groups, saline versus indomethacin.

cording to sex [22]. Overall, 29 of 196 girls (15%) and 36 of 235 boys (15%) had IVH at postnatal day 5. Girls assigned to indomethacin had the same rate of IVH as girls assigned to saline. In contrast in boys, indomethacin prophylaxis halved the incidence of IVH (9% vs. 22% in boys assigned to saline), eliminated parenchymal hemorrhage (no grade 3 or 4 IVH), and was associated with higher verbal scores at 3 to 8 years (■ Table 2.2). In addition, this effect on verbal performance in boys was independent of the agent's ability to prevent IVH.

The finding that indomethacin has an effect on both IVH and long-term cognition in VLBW boys but not girls, if confirmed, may generate new hypotheses for the sex-based prevention of injury to the developing brain. Volpe has suggested that diffuse extensive high signal intensity lesions frequently found on MRI studies result from the preterm neonate's microglia being activated by fetal inflammation and consecutively destroying developing oligodendroglia cells in response to hypoxic-ischemic and recurrent inflammatory challenges [23]. The anti-inflammatory effects of indomethacin may protect the preterm brain from injury through this mechanism, and this effect may be more pronounced in male infants [24].

Prophylactic Intravenous Ibuprofen

Four randomized controlled trails (n=672) comparing prophylactic ibuprofen with placebo or no medication for the prevention of PDA in preterm infants were included in a meta-analysis [25].

The dose and duration of prophylactic intravenous ibuprofen was similar in all the studies (10 mg/kg followed by 5 mg/kg after 24 and 48 hours interval), but the age at commencement of ibuprofen varied from 2 to 24 hours. PDA at 72 hours was diagnosed as a study outcome using echocardiographic criteria in all studies. Echocardiographic criteria of a significant PDA were similar between the studies. Backup medical treatment with COX inhibitors (indomethacin or ibuprofen) was permitted in the presence of significant PDA after initial investigational administration of ibuprofen, placebo or no medication in all trials [11, 26–28].

Prophylactic use of ibuprofen significantly reduced the incidence of PDA on day 3 in the ibuprofen group (NNT 3), the need for rescue treatment with COX inhibitors (NNT 4), and the need for surgical ligation (NNT 25) (◘ Fig. 2.2). There were no statistically significant differences in mortality,

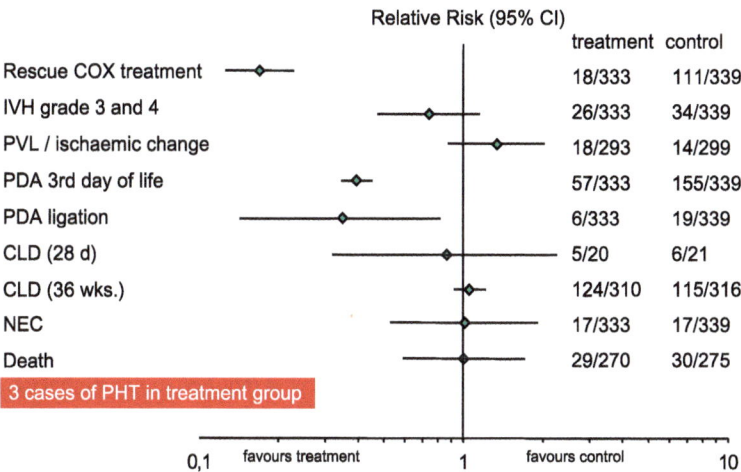

◘ **Fig. 2.2.** Meta-analysis of short-term outcomes observed in randomized controlled trials with prophylactic intravenous ibuprofen use. *COX* cyclooxygenase inhibitor; *IVH* intraventricular hemorrhage; *PVL* periventricular leukomalacia; *CLD* chronic lung disease; *NEC* necrotizing enterocolitis; *PHT* pulmonary hypertension. (Adapted from Shah and Ohlsson [25])

duration of hospitalization, grade 3 and 4 IVH, duration of mechanical ventilation, chronic lung disease (CLD) at 28 days or 36 weeks, NEC, gastrointestinal hemorrhage, intestinal perforation, time to reach full enteral feeds, retinopathy of prematurity (ROP), and sepsis between ibuprofen and placebo groups. Ibuprofen prophylaxis has a negative effect on kidney function, indicated by a statistically significant increase in the serum creatinine levels on day three of treatment in the prophylactic ibuprofen group as compared to the placebo group. The occurrence of oliguria reached borderline statistical significance. One trial (n=135) reported on three infants <1000 g who developed severe hypoxemia in the ibuprofen group. Hypoxemia was thought to be due to pulmonary hypertension, as echocardiography showed severely decreased pulmonary blood flow. Hypoxemia was responsive to inhaled nitric oxide treatment [29]. The trial was stopped prematurely due to this adverse effect. The authors postulated that this could be due to early administration of ibuprofen (<6 hours) preventing the normal fall in pulmonary vascular resistance, acidification of their ibuprofen solution causing precipitation and micro embolism in the lungs, or due to a specific effect of ibuprofen.

As the PDA had closed spontaneously by day three in 60% of the neonates in the control group prophylactic treatment would expose a large proportion of infants unnecessarily to a drug that has important side effects (mainly involving the kidneys) without conferring any important short-term benefits. Therefore, prophylactic treatment with ibuprofen is not supported by current evidence.

Until now long-term follow-up results have not been published from the trials included in the meta-analysis.

Prophylactic Ligation of the Ductus Arteriosus

One randomized controlled trial compared the effects of prophylactic surgical ligation in infants who weighed ≤1000 g and who required supplemental oxygen during the first 24 hours after birth (n=40) with a control group (n=44), in which surgery was performed only if a hemodynamically "important" PDA developed [30]. This prophylactic ligation trial by Cassady et al. is particularly interesting because it is the only randomized trial to date, in which the infants with ductal ligation were not previously exposed to a symptomatic PDA and in which the control group was not treated with a different form of

Table 2.3. Prophylactic ligation of the ductus arteriosus in infants ≤1000 g

	Control (n=44)	Prophylactic ligation (n=40)
Birth weight [g]	795 ± 98	800 ± 125
Gestation [weeks]	27.6 ± 1.5	27.4 ± 1.8
Female [%]	26 (59%)	20 (50%)
IVH (grade III/IV) [%]	23/41 (56%)	16/35 (46%)
Ductus ligation [%]	23 (52%)	38 (95%)*
Interstitial emphysema or pneumothorax [%]	19/38 (50%)	17/33 (52%)
Necrotizing enterocolitis [%]	13 (30%)	3 (8%)*
O_2 requirement at 36 weeks postmenstrual age [%]	4 (9%)	11 (28%)*
Mech. vent. at 36 weeks postmenstrual age [%]	0 (0%)	6 (15%)*
Survival beyond 35 weeks postmenstrual age [%]	19 (43%)	23 (57%)
Survival [%][†]	18 (41%)	15 (38%)

Adapted from Cassady et al. and Clyman et al. [30, 31]. Values are mean ± SD. *p<0.05 for prophylactic ligation group versus control. [†]Survival through 1 year after birth.

therapy (e.g. indomethacin). Cassady et al. concluded that early surgical closure of the ductus arteriosus reduces the risk of NEC in extremely low birth weight infants who require supplemental oxygen (3 cases in the prophylactic ligation group versus 13 in the control group, p=0.002; ◘ Table 2.3).

In recent years, the definition of BPD was changed to better reflect the degree of chronic respiratory disease in preterm infants. Clyman et al. hypothesized that the definition of BPD (defined according to the criteria of Bancalari et al.) that was used in the trial by Cassady et al. may have underestimated the true burden of CLD in their study population. The secondary analysis of the summary data sheets from the original trial by Cassady et al. revealed that although prophylactic surgical ligation of the PDA eliminates the left to right shunt, it also increases the risk of moderate/severe BPD [31]. The mechanisms underlying this increased risk are unclear. It could be due to the impact of the thoracotomy or other factors. An important caveat needs to be mentioned if one tries to extrapolate these results to present-day clinical care. The study patients in the original trial differed in many ways from today's neonatal population. They were not exposed to prenatal steroids and did not receive surfactant or indomethacin. A large proportion was also small for gestational age. In addition, changes in perinatal management, ventilatory strategies, and advances in early nutrition may limit the applicability of these findings to current neonatal care.

These results emphasize that surgical ligation should neither be used prophylactically nor as a first line treatment for a PDA, but – if at all – cautiously considered as a therapeutic option when a PDA remains hemodynamically important after failed pharmacological therapy.

Therapeutic Use of Cyclooxygenase Inhibitors for Patent Ductus Arteriosus Intervention

The meta-analysis by Ohlsson et al. on efficacy and safety of ibuprofen compared to indomethacin for closing a PDA in preterm infants has been updated recently [32]. After addition of five further studies (n=280) to the update, their review now includes twenty controlled trials involving 1092 infants. Only one study (n=136) comparing ibuprofen to placebo was identified [12], while the others compared one or several doses of ibuprofen to one or several doses of indomethacin. Among the later, seven small single center studies evaluated the use of an oral ibuprofen suspension in preterm infants below 35 weeks gestational age (n=189) [33–39]. The main outcome measure "failure rates for PDA closure with ibuprofen compared to indomethacin" was reported in nineteen studies (n=956). Data from the relevant trials found no statistically significant difference in the effectiveness of ibuprofen compared to indomethacin in closing the PDA (◻ Fig. 2.3). Furthermore, orogastric administration of ibuprofen appears as effective as the intravenous administration in closing a PDA. No statistically significant differences were found between indomethacin and ibuprofen for neonatal mortality, re-opening of the ductus arteriosus, surgical duct ligation after failed medical intervention, incidence of IVH, ROP,

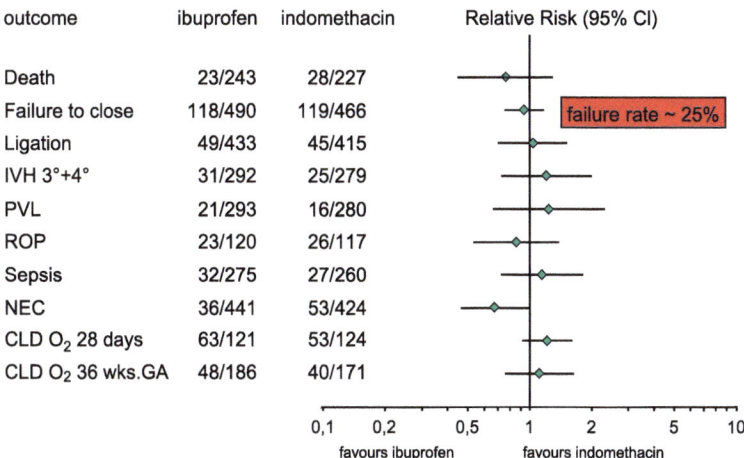

outcome	ibuprofen	indomethacin	Relative Risk (95% CI)
Death	23/243	28/227	
Failure to close	118/490	119/466	failure rate ~ 25%
Ligation	49/433	45/415	
IVH 3°+4°	31/292	25/279	
PVL	21/293	16/280	
ROP	23/120	26/117	
Sepsis	32/275	27/260	
NEC	36/441	53/424	
CLD O$_2$ 28 days	63/121	53/124	
CLD O$_2$ 36 wks.GA	48/186	40/171	

◘ Fig. 2.3. Meta-analysis of short-term outcomes observed in randomized trials comparing indomethacin and ibuprofen use for the treatment of patent ductus arteriosus in preterm infants. *IVH* intraventricular hemorrhage; *PVL* periventricular leukomalacia; *ROP* retinopathy of prematurity; *NEC* necrotizing enterocolitis; *CLD* chronic lung disease. (Adapted from Ohlsson et al. [32])

sepsis, PVL, gastrointestinal bleeding, intestinal perforation, duration of ventilator support, CLD or length of hospital stay.

Pulmonary hypertension has been observed after the prophylactic use of ibuprofen, and was also reported as adverse effect after therapeutic ibuprofen use in three infants from two trials included in this meta-analysis [12, 40]. Another potential side effect of ibuprofen is a decreased bilirubin-albumin binding capacity [41]. However, published data on bilirubin toxicity from prospective randomized trials are not available.

Compared with indomethacin, ibuprofen causes fewer transient adverse effects on the renal function and reduces the risk of NEC (15 studies [n=865]; typical RR 0.68 [95% CI 0.47, 0.99]; p=0.04; NNT 25). No individual study found a significant difference in the rates of NEC. These two outcomes were the only clinical findings favoring ibuprofen.

Besides, ibuprofen enhances cerebral autoregulation without affecting cerebral blood flow, or cerebral metabolism in piglets [42, 43]. Ibuprofen has been also shown to have some neuroprotective effects in animal models [44, 45].

Whether these favorable biochemical and physiological data on ibuprofen confer any important long-term advantages on development or not is unknown. Until now, randomized controlled trials evaluating the effect of ibuprofen compared to indomethacin on longer-term outcomes in infants with PDA are lacking.

Neurodevelopmental Outcome After Therapeutic Use of Cyclooxygenase Inhibitors

The fact that no data on neurodevelopmental follow-up after therapeutic use have been published for either of the two COX inhibitors inspired us to evaluate whether neurological outcome differed between infants treated with ibuprofen or indomethacin in our own patient cohort. In a retrospective study, we analysed closure rates, short-term outcome parameters and neurodevelopmental results at two years corrected age of 182 VLBW infants undergoing COX inhibitor treatment (89 indomethacin and 93 ibuprofen) for a haemodynamically significant PDA (hsPDA) in the Department of Neonatology, Charité Campus Virchow-Klinikum, Berlin, Germany between 1998 and 2003 (◘ Fig. 2.4) [46]. Altogether 617 VLBW infants were treated in our unit during the study period. Two-year outcome data were available in 141 of the 182 infants with a PDA that were considered to require intervention. The flaws and disadvantages of the historical design are partly counterbalanced by strict therapy standards and staff that remained largely unchanged during the study period as well as a low rate of infants lost to follow-up. They are also mitigated by the fact that, with the exception of a change in preferred drug treatment in 2001, general management strategies for PDA did not undergo significant changes at our hospital in the specified time period, leading us to conclude that their effect on our data is inconsequential. In our department COX inhibitor treatment is only initiated in VLBW infants with a hsPDA. A PDA with left-to-right shunt was considered hemodynamically significant if (i) a respiratory set back with a supplemental oxygen requirement >30% and/or mechanical ventilation, (ii) a LA/Ao ratio ≥1.4 in the echocardiogram and/or (iii) a decreased enddiastolic flow in the anterior cerebral artery with a resistance index ≥0.85 in the cerebral ultrasound was present. From January 1998 to March 2001 infants received indomethacin, starting with three doses of 0.2 mg/kg in 12 hour intervals followed by daily maintenance doses of 0.1 mg/kg for a maximum of 6 days. From April 2001 to December 2003 ibuprofen (Pedea®) with the standard dose regimen of 10–5–5 mg/kg at 24 hour inter-

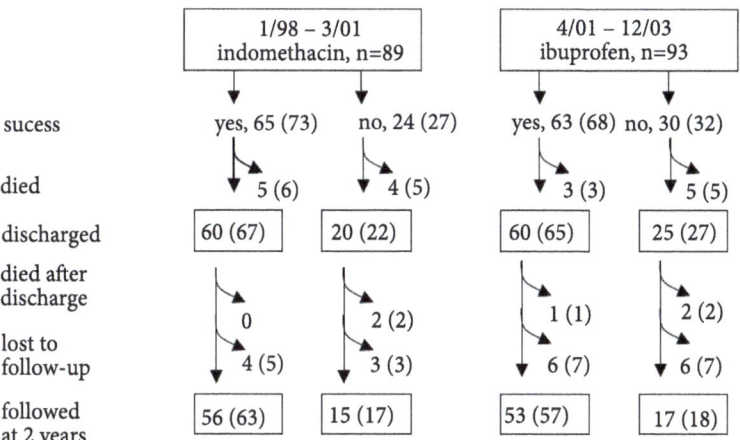

■ **Fig. 2.4.** Patient flow after diagnosis of a hemodynamically significant PDA. Numbers are displayed as n (%). Upper boxes display study periods and COX inhibitor therapy groups. Success is defined as successful pharmacological PDA closure. All infants with failed pharmacological PDA closure (with the exception of two from the ibuprofen group who died before ligation) received surgical ligation. Lower boxes display numbers of infants with complete follow-up data at 24 months corrected age

vals was used to treat hsPDA. Successful response to COX inhibitor treatment was defined as absent ductal shunt flow at 24–48 hours after therapy, all other cases were defined as COX inhibitor treatment failure. Ligation by clip was performed as a rescue therapy after failure of pharmacological treatment in ventilated infants by two cardiosurgeons directly in the NICU in a mean operation time of 20–30 min through a left lateral thoracotomy. Follow-up examinations were done on infants at two years corrected age in our outpatient clinic by a neonatologist specialized in neurodevelopmental testing and a child psychologist. Neurodevelopmental status was evaluated using Griffiths score subscales for motor performance, personal and social behavior, hearing and speech ability, hand coordination and cognition until March 2005. A test result below 88 points (>2 SD, mean 22 months corrected age = 98 points, range 96–112 points) indicates severe impairment [47]. From January 2004 neurodevelopmental testing was evaluated with the Bayley Scales II of Infant Development for cognitive, social, speech and gross and fine motor skills. A result of less than 70 points (>2 SD, mean 24 months corrected age = 100 points,

Table 2.4. Baseline data of infants before cyclooxygenase inhibitor treatment

	Indomethacin (n=89)	Ibuprofen (n=93)	p
Birthweight [g]	845 (730–1072)	850 (717–1127)	n.s.
GA [wks.d]	26.0 (25.0–28.0)	26.2 (25.0–27.6)	n.s.
CRIB score	6 (2–9)	5 (3–8)	n.s.
Female, n [%]	44 (49)	32 (34)	0.04
Inborn, n [%]	80 (90)	84 (90)	n.s.
Antenatal steroids, n [%]	62 (70)	62 (67)	n.s.
RDS > grade 2, n [%]	36 (40)	34 (37)	n.s.
Surfactant therapy, n [%]	67 (75)	68 (73)	n.s.
Maximum FiO$_2$	0.6 (0.3–0.8)	0.44 (0.32–0.8)	n.s.
Mechanical ventilation, n [%]	54 (62)	52 (57)	n.s.
Age at first intervention [d]	4 (3–7)	3 (2–6)	n.s.

Median and quartiles are displayed, if not otherwise indicated. *GA* gestational age; *CRIB* critical risk index for babies; *RDS* respiratory distress syndrome; *FiO$_2$* fraction of inspired oxygen.

range 85–115 points) indicates severe impairment [48]. The change from Griffiths DQ to Bayley scales for neurodevelopmental testing in accordance with international standards during the study period is one limitation of our study. Since the numerical scores of the two test sets are not equivalent, it is not possible to compare median test results directly. No comparative study of both tests has been done for preterm infants. It has, however, been demonstrated in other patient populations that both tests can be used interchangeably [49, 50]. In the period where both test methods were used simultaneously, the outcome of 11 infants was equally categorized as either normal (7 infants) or poor (4 infants). The fact that all follow-up examinations were performed by the same examiners during the entire study period supports the reliability of our follow-up analysis despite the use of two different tests.

□ Table 2.5. Short-term outcome of infants after PDA intervention

	Indomethacin (n=89)	Ibuprofen (n=93)	COX-inhibitor treatment failure (n=54)
Birthweight [g]	845 (730–1072)	850 (717–1127)	750* (665–881)
GA [wks.d]	26.0 (25.0–28.0)	26.2 (25.0–27.6)	25.0* (24.3–26.5)
CRIB score	6 (2–9)	5 (3–8)	7 (4–10)*
Survivors, n [%]	80 (90)	85 (91)	45 (83)*
IVH > 2°, n [%]	10 (11)	9 (10)	5 (10)
CLD (28 d), n [%]	49 (61)	55 (65)	43 (96)*
CLD (36 wks.), n [%]	31 (35)	27 (29)	31 (68)*
PVL, n [%]	7 (8)	6 (7)	6 (13)
ROP > 2°, n [%]	9 (10)	5 (5)	9 (20)*
NEC, n [%]	10 (11)	11 (12)	5 (10)
Hospitalization days	89 (72–106)	76 (60–96)	101 (82–131)*
COX-treatment failure, n [%]	24 (27)	30 (32)	

Median and quartiles are displayed, if not otherwise indicated. *p<0.05 for COX-inhibitor treatment failure group versus success. *GA* gestational age; *CRIB* critical risk index for babies; *IVH* intraventricular hemorrhage; *CLD* chronic lung disease; *PVL* periventricular leukomalacia; *ROP* retinopathy of prematurity; *NEC* necrotizing enterocolitis; *COX* cyclooxygenase inhibitor.

Comparison of infants who were treated with ibuprofen or indomethacin revealed no differences in their baseline clinical profile apart from a higher number of female individuals in the indomethacin group (□ Table 2.4). No differences were found in perinatal and early and late morbidity data (□ Table 2.5). The number of infants with therapy related oliguria (indomethacin 3 and ibuprofen 1) was small in both groups. PDA closure rates were alike

Table 2.6. Neurodevelopmental results of infants after PDA intervention

	Indo-methacin (n=89)	Ibuprofen (n=93)	COX-inhibitor treatment failure (n=54)
Survivors follow-up, n [%]	78 (88)	82 (88)	41 (76)
Follow-up complete, n [%)	71 (91)	70 (85)	32 (78)
Hearing threshold >35dB, n [%]	7 (10)	7 (10)	3 (9)
EMPP 12 months >4, n [%|	12 (17)	9 (13)	9 (28)
Griffiths' DQ 22 months	92 (84–97)	98 (88–105)	93 (90–97)
Bayley MDI 24 months	–	87 (72–98)	80 (49–87)
Griffiths' 22 months <88 or Bayley 24 months <70, n [%]	23 (32)	15 (22)	7 (22)
Free walking at 2 years, n [%]	67 (94)	67 (96)	30 (94)
Composite poor outcome, n [%]	27 (38)	19 (28)	8 (25)

Only data of infants with complete follow-up data are shown. A composite poor outcome was defined as the infant's exhibiting one or more of the following at a corrected age of two years: no free walking, Griffiths DQ score of less than 88, Bayley MDI score of less than 70, bilateral blindness, or bilateral hearing impairment requiring amplification. Median and quartiles are displayed, if not otherwise indicated. *EMPP* early motor pattern profile; *DQ* developmental quotient; *MDI* mental developmental index.

in both groups (Table 2.5). An efficacy of 70% closure rate after COX-inhibitor therapy leaves room for improvement, as a higher success rate would probably lower ligation rate and hence could lead to better outcome results. Prolongation of COX-inhibitor therapy as well as the escalation of doses has been discussed and investigated recently [51–53]. The prolonged indomethacin protocol used in our study did not improve the rate of successful PDA closure in comparison to the ibuprofen group treated with the standard dosing.

The different pharmacological profiles and the varied undesirable side effects associated with each drug, did not seem to have relevant impact on neurodevelopmental outcome at two years in our study population of VLBW infants treated for a hsPDA (◘ Table 2.6). Since we detected no significant differences in mortality or severely impaired neurodevelopmental outcome at two years between the two COX-inhibitor therapy groups, this retrospective data analysis does not indicate whether indomethacin or ibuprofen is preferable for the pharmacological therapy of a PDA.

Surgical Ligation of Patent Ductus Arteriosus After Failed Pharmacological Intervention

The question of the impact of PDA ligation in preterm infants has been thoroughly discussed recently. Following a retrospective data analysis on the short-term complications of indomethacin and surgical treatment for PDA performed over a 12 year period from 1987 until 1998, we proposed that surgical ligation should be reserved for infants not responding to pharmacological PDA closure (◘ Table 2.7) [54]. Besides adverse events related to the surgical procedure itself, PDA ligation has been shown to be associated with neonatal morbidities such as BPD, ROP and neurosensory impairment in extremely low birth weight (ELBW) infants [55, 56].

With our current study, we aimed to add further information to this discussion by a detailed data analysis of our hsPDA patient population (◘ Fig. 2.4) [46]. COX-inhibitor treatment was not successful in 54 infants (30%). These infants, except two who died before ligation could be performed, received ligation as a rescue therapy. These infants were significantly more premature and smaller, had worse CRIB scores and were at higher risk for death before 24 months corrected age (mortality 17%; ◘ Table 2.5). The data revealed major differences between the infants with successful COX-inhibitor therapy and those in whom therapy failed with respect to early follow-up data. In the therapy failure group rates of BPD and ROP were higher, the hospitalization period longer (◘ Table 2.5). No differences were found for rates of IVH, PVL and NEC. Not surprisingly, more infants in the therapy failure group were mechanically ventilated, given that respiratory setback (reintubation, FiO_2 >30%) was one criteria for the diagnosis of a hsPDA. Our echocardiographic data showed equal hemodynamic stress by PDA before intervention (maxi-

Table 2.7. Clinical profile of VLBW infants before PDA intervention and treatment complications

	Indomethacin (n=67)	Surgery (n=55)	Indomethacin and surgery (n=34)
Birth weight [g]	910 (525/1480)	760 (540/1250)	885 (578/1450)
GA [weeks/days]	26.4 (24.0/34.0)	26.0 (23.2/31.0)	26.1 (24.1/30.0)
Male, n [%]	31 (46)	25 (46)	17 (50)
CRIB score	8.5 (1/20)	11 (1/20)	10 (0/20)
IVH > grade 2, n [%]	7 (10)	16 (29)	4 (12)
NEC, n [%]	5 (7)	1 (2)	2 (6)
Age at intervention [days]	8 (2/21)	11 (4/27)	9 (4/23)[a] 17.5 (6/54)[b]
Tension pneumothorax	0	5	0
Pneumoperitoneum	0	1	0
Intraoperative bleeding	0	2	0
Pulmonary hemorrhage	0	1	0
Phrenic palsy	0	1	0
Wound infection	0	2	0

Clinical profile of infants before PDA intervention (upper part) and complications and adverse events after PDA intervention (lower part). Values are median (range) or numbers (%), [a]before Indomethacin therapy, [b]before surgery. *GA* gestational age; *CRIB* critical risk index for babies; *IVH* intraventricular hemorrhage; *NEC* necrotizing enterocolitis.

mum PDA diameter, number of infants with PDA diameter >1.5 mm, left atrium to aortic root ratio ≥1.4 and/or resistance index ≥0.85) in both groups. PDA duration was longer in the therapy failure group supposedly because of the time needed to arrange for surgical ligation. The evident differences in clinical data of the therapy failure compared to the success group led to the expectation that neurodevelopmental outcome might differ as well, but surprisingly, we saw no difference in neurodevelopmental test results between the surviving infants with ligation and the survivors with successful pharmacological closure of the PDA at 24 months corrected age (◘ Table 2.6). This result was not due to death of the most severely impaired infants during their second year of life. All together 5 infants died during the follow-up period, one in the therapy success group (persistent pulmonary hypertension) and 4 infants in the therapy failure group (1 diagnosis unknown, 2 infants with unknown syndrome, and 1 SIDS). The inclusion of death into a composite variable of "poor outcome" did not result in a significant difference between the treatment success and the treatment failure groups despite the fact that treatment failure infants were lighter and had higher CRIB scores at birth. Our findings are in agreement with reports that birth weight and CRIB score have a higher predictive power for neonatal morbidity and mortality than for neurodevelopmental outcome [57]. To rule out a bias due to the change in the use of the Griffiths to the Bayley scales during the study period, we analyzed the data subsets of each test separately. In the Griffiths DQ 79 infants of the treatment success group (median 92 points; Q 1/3: 83/100) and 23 infants of the treatment failure group (median 92 points; Q 1/3: 89/96, p>0.16) were tested at 22 months. In the Bayley test 32 infants of the treatment success group (median 90 points; Q 1/3: 75/99) and 13 infants of the treatment failure group (median 80 points; Q 1/3: 49/87, p>0.06) were tested at 24 months. No differences were found in hearing and walking ability or composite poor outcome at 24 months corrected age (◘ Table 2.6).

In our study, failed PDA closure following COX-inhibitor therapy was associated with prematurity, neonatal morbidity and mortality, but not with poor neurodevelopmental outcome of the surviving infants at two years corrected age. Both the Schmidt and Clyman groups have published prospective studies on that issue [55, 56]. The perinatal data of their and our study have consistently shown that the smallest, most premature infants are those that require surgical ligation after failed PDA closure by COX-inhibitor therapy. In a retrospective study Noori's group has shown that the failure of ductal closure is associated with an increase in mortality in very preterm infants [58]. Failed PDA closure is associated with morbidity represented by prolonged hospitalization and higher mortality in our study population as well.

In the therapy failure group the follow-up recall rate is significantly lower than in the success group, 78% vs. 92% respectively. Poor outcome is associ-

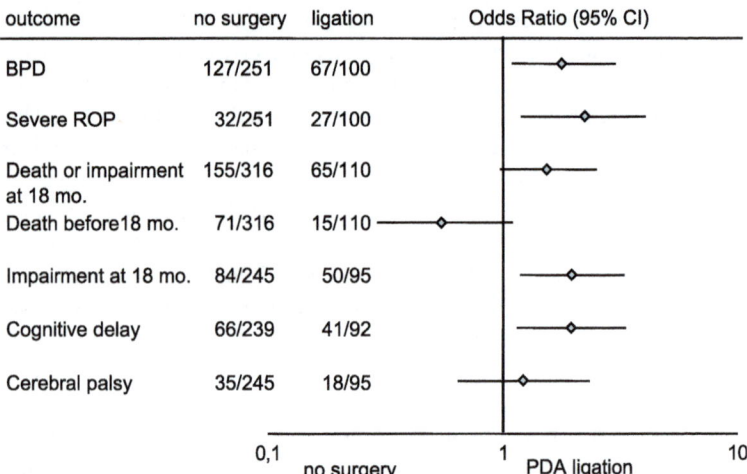

◘ Fig. 2.5. Meta-analysis of outcome at 18 months corrected age after no surgery versus PDA ligation. (Adapted from Kabra et al. [56])

ated with parental noncompliance for different reasons, and it is therefore conceivable that the follow-up results in the treatment failure group may have been worse if the follow-up rate in this group had been higher, as the Clyman work has shown [55]. Additionally, an extended follow-up assessment at 5 years corrected age will contribute to this question and might identify significant differences that are not apparent at two years. It is impossible to separately evaluate the effect of surgical ligation and perinatal morbidity on the outcome of preterm infants in retrospective analyses. The group of Schmidt found that surgical PDA ligation in ELBW infants is associated with BPD, ROP and neurosensory impairment and suspected that ligation was a cause of a poor outcome at 18 months corrected age (◘ Fig. 2.5) [56]. However, the meta-analysis of Fowlie and Davis did not show improved neurodevelopmental outcome despite a reduction in the rate of ligation in ELBW infants with prophylactic indomethacin therapy [13]. We also found a significantly higher rate of BPD and ROP in infants who underwent ligation after failed pharmacological PDA intervention. The Clyman group with a study population twice as large as ours demonstrated no effect of surgical ligation on neurodevelopmental impairment, but showed an independent effect on CLP [55]. We agree with the Brooks group that a randomized controlled trial of surgical PDA ligation after failed pharmacological treatment is required to clarify the role of this intervention on neurodevelopmental outcome in VLBW infants [59].

Conclusions and Perspectives

Depending on individual clinical circumstances and personal preferences, there may be a role for prophylactic indomethacin in some infants on some neonatal units, e.g. units without access to cardiac surgery. Although data are available on long-term neurodevelopmental outcome up to the age of 18 months or two years in many children after prophylactic indomethacin, continuing follow-up of these children is justified as more subtle differences in later childhood/adulthood may become apparent. Ibuprofen is as effective as indomethacin in closing a PDA and causes fewer transient adverse effects. To decide whether ibuprofen or indomethacin is the drug of choice for closing a PDA follow-up studies after random allocation to either drug are necessary – and preferably should provide follow-up data up to the age of school entry. The poor long-term results seen after surgical ligation should not lead to abandoning surgery as a treatment for a PDA, but they should lead to greater caution in considering the therapeutic alternatives when a hemodynamically important PDA is present.

Further research efforts should address dilemmas that remain: the optimal dosage regimen has yet to be determined and the optimal target population in terms of birth weight, gestational age and perhaps even illness severity needs to be identified more clearly. Assessment of long-term outcomes is mandatory for any new trial.

References

1. Valls ISA, Carnielli V, Claris O et al. (2008) EuroNeoStat: a European information system on the outcomes of care for very-low-birth-weight infants (<1500 g). Z Geburtshilfe Neonatol 212: 116–118
2. Hack M, Friedman H, Fanaroff AA (1996) Outcomes of extremely low birth weight infants. Pediatrics 98: 931–937
3. Hack M (2007) Survival and neurodevelopmental outcomes of preterm infants. J Pediatr Gastroenterol Nutr 45 (Suppl 3): S141–142

2

4. Hack M (2009) Adult outcomes of preterm children. J Dev Behav Pediatr 30: 460–470

5. Hack M, Wright LL, Shankaran S et al. (1995) Very-low-birth-weight outcomes of the National Institute of Child Health and Human Development Neonatal Network, November 1989 to October 1990. Am J Obstet Gynecol 172: 457–464

6. Bhushan V, Paneth N, Kiely JL (1993) Impact of improved survival of very low birth weight infants on recent secular trends in the prevalence of cerebral palsy. Pediatrics 91: 1094–1100

7. McCarton CM, Brooks-Gunn J, Wallace IF et al. (1997) Results at age 8 years of early intervention for low-birth-weight premature infants. The Infant Health and Development Program. JAMA 277: 126–132

8. Klebanov PK, Brooks-Gunn J, McCormick MC (1994) School achievement and failure in very low birth weight children. J Dev Behav Pediatr 15: 248–256

9. Tyson JE, Parikh NA, Langer J, Green C, Higgins RD (2008) Intensive care for extreme prematurity-moving beyond gestational age. N Engl J Med 358: 1672–1681

10. The Vermont-Oxford Trials Network (1993) Very low birth weight outcomes for 1990. Investigators of the Vermont-Oxford Trials Network Database Project. Pediatrics 91: 540–545

11. Van Overmeire B, Allegaert K, Casaer A et al. (2004) Prophylactic ibuprofen in premature infants: a multicentre, randomised, double-blind, placebo-controlled trial. Lancet 364: 1945–1949

12. Aranda JV, Clyman R, Cox B et al. (2009) A randomized, double-blind, placebo-controlled trial on intravenous ibuprofen L-lysine for the early closure of nonsymptomatic patent ductus arteriosus within 72 hours of birth in extremely low-birth-weight infants. Am J Perinatol 26: 235–245

13. Fowlie PW, Davis PG (2002) Prophylactic intravenous indomethacin for preventing mortality and morbidity in preterm infants. Cochrane Database Syst Rev: CD000174

14. Fowlie PW, Davis PG (2003) Prophylactic indomethacin for preterm infants: a systematic review and meta-analysis. Arch Dis Child Fetal Neonatal Ed 88: F464–466

15. Ment LR, Oh W, Ehrenkranz RA et al. (1994) Low-dose indomethacin and prevention of intraventricular hemorrhage: a multicenter randomized trial. Pediatrics 93: 543–550

16. Schmidt B, Davis P, Moddemann D et al. (2001) Long-term effects of indomethacin prophylaxis in extremely-low-birth-weight infants. N Engl J Med 344: 1966–1972

17. Bandstra ES, Montalvo BM, Goldberg RN et al. (1988) Prophylactic indomethacin for prevention of intraventricular hemorrhage in premature infants. Pediatrics 82: 533–542

18. Ment LR, Vohr B, Oh W et al. (1996) Neurodevelopmental outcome at 36 months' corrected age of preterm infants in the Multicenter Indomethacin Intraventricular Hemorrhage Prevention Trial. Pediatrics 98: 714–718

19. Ment LR, Vohr B, Allan W et al. (2000) Outcome of children in the indomethacin intraventricular hemorrhage prevention trial. Pediatrics 105: 485–491

20. Vohr BR, Allan WC, Westerveld M et al. (2003) School-age outcomes of very low birth weight infants in the indomethacin intraventricular hemorrhage prevention trial. Pediatrics 111: e340–346

21. Geary GG, Krause DN, Duckles SP (2000) Gonadal hormones affect diameter of male rat cerebral arteries through endothelium-dependent mechanisms. Am J Physiol Heart Circ Physiol 279: H610–618

22. Ment LR, Vohr BR, Makuch RW et al. (2004) Prevention of intraventricular hemorrhage by indomethacin in male preterm infants. J Pediatr 145: 832–834

23. Volpe JJ (2003) Cerebral white matter injury of the premature infant-more common than you think. Pediatrics 112: 176–180

24. Monje ML, Toda H, Palmer TD (2003) Inflammatory blockade restores adult hippocampal neurogenesis. Science 302: 1760–1765

25. Shah SS, Ohlsson A (2006) Ibuprofen for the prevention of patent ductus arteriosus in preterm and/or low birth weight infants. Cochrane Database Syst Rev: CD004213

26. Dani C, Bertini G, Reali MF et al. (2000) Prophylaxis of patent ductus arteriosus with ibuprofen in preterm infants. Acta Paediatr 89: 1369–1374

27. De Carolis MP, Romagnoli C, Polimeni V et al. (2000) Prophylactic ibuprofen therapy of patent ductus arteriosus in preterm infants. Eur J Pediatr 159: 364–368

28. Gournay V, Roze JC, Kuster A et al. (2004) Prophylactic ibuprofen versus placebo in very premature infants: a randomised, double-blind, placebo-controlled trial. Lancet 364: 1939–1944

29. Gournay V, Savagner C, Thiriez G, Kuster A, Roze JC (2002) Pulmonary hypertension after ibuprofen prophylaxis in very preterm infants. Lancet 359: 1486–1488

30. Cassady G, Crouse DT, Kirklin JW et al. (1989) A randomized, controlled trial of very early prophylactic ligation of the ductus arteriosus in babies who weighed 1000 g or less at birth. N Engl J Med 320: 1511–1516

31. Clyman R, Cassady G, Kirklin JK, Collins M, Philips JB 3rd (2009) The role of patent ductus arteriosus ligation in bronchopulmonary dysplasia: reexamining a randomized controlled trial. J Pediatr 154: 873–876

32. Ohlsson A, Walia R, Shah SS (2010) Ibuprofen for the treatment of patent ductus arteriosus in preterm and/or low birth weight infants. Cochrane Database Syst Rev: CD003481

33. Aly H, Lotfy W, Badrawi N, Ghawas M, Abdel-Meguid IE, Hammad TA (2007) Oral Ibuprofen and ductus arteriosus in premature infants: a randomized pilot study. Am J Perinatol 24: 267–270

34. Chotigeat U, Jirapapa K, Layangkool T (2003) A comparison of oral ibuprofen and intravenous indomethacin for closure of patent ductus arteriosus in preterm infants. J Med Assoc Thai 86 (Suppl 3): S563–569

35. Salama H, Alsisi A, Al-Rifai H et al. (2008) A randomized controlled trial on the use of oral ibuprofen to close patent ductus arteriosus in premature infants. J Neonat-Perinat Med 1: 153–158

36. Supapannachart S, Limrungsikul A, Khowsathit P (2002) Oral ibuprofen and indomethacin for treatment of patent ductus arteriosus in premature infants: a randomized trial at Ramathibodi Hospital. J Med Assoc Thai 85 (Suppl 4): S1252–1258

37. Akisu M, Ozyurek AR, Dorak C, Parlar A, Kultursay N (2001) Enteral ibuprofen versus indomethacin in the treatment of patent ductus arteriosus in preterm newborn infants [Premature bebeklerde patent duktus arteriozusun tedavisinde enteral ibuprofen ve indometazinin etkinligi ve guvenilirligi]. Cocuk Sagligi ve Hastaliklari Dergisi 44: 56–60

38. Fakhraee SH, Badiee Z, Mojtahedzadeh S, Kazemian M, Kelishadi R (2007) Comparison of oral ibuprofen and indomethacin therapy for patent ductus arteriosus in preterm infants. Chinese Journal of Contemporary Pediatrics 9: 399–403

39. Pourarian S, Pishva N, Madani A, Rastegari M (2008) Comparison of oral ibuprofen and indomethacin on closure of patent ductus arteriosus in preterm infants. Eastern Mediterranean Health Journal 14: 360–365

40. Adamska E, Helwich E, Rutkowska M, Zacharska E, Piotrowska A (2005) Comparison of the efficacy of ibuprofen and indomethacin in the treatment of patent ductus arteriosus in prematurely born infants [Porownanie ibuprofenu i indometacyny w leczeniu przetrwalego przewodu tetniczego u noworodkow urodzonych przedwczesnie]. Medycyna wieku rozwojowego 9: 335–354

41. Ahlfors CE (2004) Effect of ibuprofen on bilirubin-albumin binding. J Pediatr 144: 386–388

42. Chemtob S, Beharry K, Barna T, Varma DR, Aranda JV (1991) Differences in the effects in the newborn piglet of various nonsteroidal antiinflammatory drugs on cerebral blood flow but not on cerebrovascular prostaglandins. Pediatr Res 30: 106–111

43. Hardy P, Peri KG, Lahaie I, Varma DR, Chemtob S (1996) Increased nitric oxide synthesis and action preclude choroidal vasoconstriction to hyperoxia in newborn pigs. Circ Res 79: 504–511

44. Chemtob S, Beharry K, Rex J, Varma DR, Aranda JV (1990) Prostanoids determine the range of cerebral blood flow autoregulation of newborn piglets. Stroke 21: 777–784

45. Pellicer A, Aparicio M, Cabanas F, Valverde E, Quero J, Stiris TA (1999) Effect of the cyclooxygenase blocker ibuprofen on cerebral blood volume and cerebral blood flow during normocarbia and hypercarbia in newborn piglets. Acta Paediatr 88: 82–88

46. Rheinlaender C, Helfenstein D, Pees C et al. (2010) Neurodevelopmental outcome after COX inhibitor treatment for patent ductus arteriosus. Early Hum Dev 86: 87–92

47. Brandt I, Sticker E. Griffith (2001) Entwicklungsskalen (GES) zur Beurteilung der Entwicklung in den ersten beiden Lebensjahren. 2. Aufl. Beltz Test-GmbH, Göttingen

48. Bayley N (1999) Bayley scales of infant development (Bsid-II). 3rd edn. Pearson Psychcorp, Sydney

49. Beail N (1985) A comparative study of profoundly multiply handicapped children's scores on the Bayley and the Griffiths developmental scales. Child Care Health Dev 11: 31–36

50. Ramsay M, Fitzhardinge PM (1977) A comparative study of two developmental scales: the Bayley and the Griffiths. Early Hum Dev 1: 151–157

51. Sperandio M, Beedgen B, Feneberg R et al. (2005) Effectiveness and side effects of an escalating, stepwise approach to indomethacin treatment for symptomatic patent ductus arteriosus in premature infants below 33 weeks of gestation. Pediatrics 116: 1361–1366

52. Hirt D, Van Overmeire B, Treluyer JM et al. (2008) An optimized ibuprofen dosing scheme for preterm neonates with patent ductus arteriosus, based on a population pharmacokinetic and pharmacodynamic study. Br J Clin Pharmacol 65: 629–636

53. Jegatheesan P, Ianus V, Buchh B et al. (2008) Increased indomethacin dosing for persistent patent ductus arteriosus in preterm infants: a multicenter, randomized, controlled trial. J Pediatr 153: 183–189

54. Koehne PS, Bein G, Alexi-Meskhishvili V, Weng Y, Buhrer C, Obladen M (2001) Patent ductus arteriosus in very low birthweight infants: complications of pharmacological and surgical treatment. J Perinat Med 29: 327–334

55. Chorne N, Leonard C, Piecuch R, Clyman RI (2007) Patent ductus arteriosus and its treatment as risk factors for neonatal and neurodevelopmental morbidity. Pediatrics 119: 1165–1174

56. Kabra NS, Schmidt B, Roberts RS, Doyle LW, Papile L, Fanaroff A (2007) Neurosensory impairment after surgical closure of patent ductus arteriosus in extremely low birth weight infants: results from the Trial of Indomethacin Prophylaxis in Preterms. J Pediatr 150: 229–234, 34 e1

57. Buhrer C, Grimmer I, Metze B, Obladen M (2000) The CRIB (Clinical Risk Index for Babies) score and neurodevelopmental impairment at one year corrected age in very low birth weight infants. Intensive Care Med 26: 325–329

58. Noori S, McCoy M, Friedlich P et al. (2009) Failure of ductus arteriosus closure is associated with increased mortality in preterm infants. Pediatrics 123: e138–144

59. Brooks JM, Travadi JN, Patole SK, Doherty DA, Simmer K (2005) Is surgical ligation of patent ductus arteriosus necessary? The Western Australian experience of conservative management. Arch Dis Child Fetal Neonatal Ed 90: F235–239

Echocardiographic Assessment of the Patent Ductus Arteriosus in the Preterm Infant

N. Evans

Introduction

Opinion on the importance of the preterm persistent ductus arteriosus (PDA) has swung between being viewed as the cause of most preterm adverse outcomes to being viewed as an innocent physiological bystander. The former view derives from observational studies of the pathophysiology of the PDA [1, 2] and statistical associations with adverse outcomes [3]. The "innocent bystander" view derives from the amalgamation of historically and methodologically diverse randomised trials [4–6]. These reviews show little evidence of consistent effect on outcomes of treating PDA leading to conclusions that if treating makes no difference to outcomes then PDA may not be pathological for the preterm infant. While this is one possible conclusion, there are other equally valid ones, specifically whether we have really understood what is going wrong and whether we have asked the treatment questions in the correct way? While systematic review is good at defining the limits of our understanding, it paints pictures with too broad a brush to allow definition of which questions should be asked and how we should ask them. For that there is no substitute for looking at the babies and their ducts so we can understand what is physiological and what is pathological. To do this you need ultrasound.

Doppler Ultrasound

In the simplest terms, ultrasounds reflect off solid or liquid interfaces of different density to allow definition of structure. In the heart, this is the interface between muscle, fibre and blood. Projection of these structures against time allows definition of movement, both of the structures themselves but also relative to other structures. Such is the essence of M-mode and two-dimensional imaging. The Doppler principle can be applied to ultrasounds because they change frequency as they reflect off moving objects. The direction of change in frequency depends on the direction of movement of the object. Movement towards the transmission source increases frequency, movement away decreases the frequency. This frequency shift is directly proportional to the velocity of the moving object as long as the direction of movement is within 20 degrees of straight towards or straight away from the transmission source. So when this is applied to blood moving in the heart and blood vessels, the various types of Doppler allow determination of two factors; direction of blood flow and velocity of that flow. Colour Doppler maps this directional velocity information on the 2D image, with blood flow towards the transducer coded red and away from the transducer coded blue.

So Doppler ultrasound allows the direct imaging of the ductus to determine patency and degree of constriction. This is aided by colour Doppler mapping which confirms the presence and direction of any shunt and the degree of constriction. Pulsed Doppler can be used to more accurately measure the pattern and velocity of the shunt as well as assessing disturbance to the pattern of blood flow, particularly diastolic flow, in the major vessels either side of the duct. Put another way, Doppler ultrasound assessment of the ductus can answer several questions:

1. Is the ductus patent?
2. If the ductus is patent, how wide is it or, in other words, how well has it constricted?
3. What is the direction and velocity of the shunt?
4. What is the significance of the shunt and what is the impact on the systemic and pulmonary circulation?
5. Finally it allows prediction of closure, either spontaneously or in response to therapeutic intervention.

Is the Ductus Arteriosus Patent?

The resolution of modern ultrasound is such that indirect echocardiographic methods for assessing ductal patency have been rendered largely obsolete, though as described below, they may add information on the significance of a ductal shunt. Occasionally indirect markers can be useful in chronically ventilated babies where over inflation of the lungs can restrict the echocardiographic window for direct imaging. Determining ductal patency should involve direct imaging. The ductus leaves the main pulmonary artery (MPA) at its junction with the left pulmonary artery (LPA). This left sided offset of the duct reflects its course into the left sided descending aorta. The ductus continues in the same posterior direction as the MPA to describe an arch into the descending aorta (■ Fig. 3.1). Imaging involves placing the transducer over the ductus in a left sided high parasternal position and aligning the beam in a true sagittal plane to follow the true antero-posterior direction of the ductal course. If the user initially aligns the image down the body of the MPA and then angles

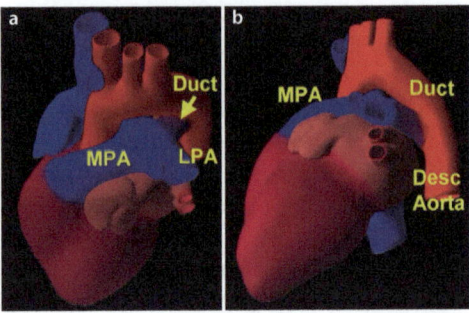

◘ **Fig. 3.1a,b.** Shows the anatomical relationships of the ductus with the view from above (a) showing how the ductus is a slightly left sided continuation of the main pulmonary artery which describes an arch into the descending aorta as seen from the left side in (b)

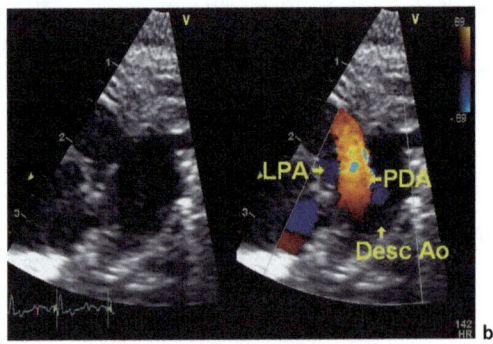

◘ **Fig. 3.2a,b.** Shows the true saggital ductal cut with a widely patent duct apparent on 2D imaging (a) and on colour Doppler (b) with the red left to right ductal shunt contrasting with the blue streams in the left pulmonary artery and descending aorta

the beam slightly to the left to image the root of the LPA (seen as a diverticulum), the course of the ductus will be seen just superior to the root of the LPA (◘ Fig. 3.2).

A ductus that is widely patent will be readily apparent on 2D imaging but confirmation of patency requires colour Doppler to show the shunt of blood through the duct (◘ Fig. 3.2). The common left-to-right shunt travelling towards the transducer codes in red and contrasts strongly with the streams in the LPA and descending aorta which code blue. Care needs to be taken that the less common right to left shunt is not missed as this will code blue like the adjacent streams so gets easily overlooked.

How Wide is the Ductus Arteriosus?

The fetal ductus arteriosus is a large vessel not much smaller than the MPA reflecting the fact that it carries 90–95% of the cardiac output. In the early postnatal period almost all babies will show some degree of constriction from this fetal size. In healthy term babies, this early constriction is universal, powerful and often occurs along the length of the ductus, in preterm babies it is more variable as will be discussed below. The constriction can be quite localised, usually at the pulmonary end of the ductus, so it is important to image the ductus along its length to measure the minimum size, e.g site of maximum constriction.

These differences in ductal constriction are readily apparent on colour Doppler and 2D imaging (◘ Fig. 3.3). With high-resolution equipment and a good ultrasound window this can be measured just using 2D imaging but the course of the duct means that the ultrasound beams hit the ductal walls at near to 180° so the edge resolution is often not good. As a result, ductal diameter or width is often measured using the colour Doppler stream. This requires

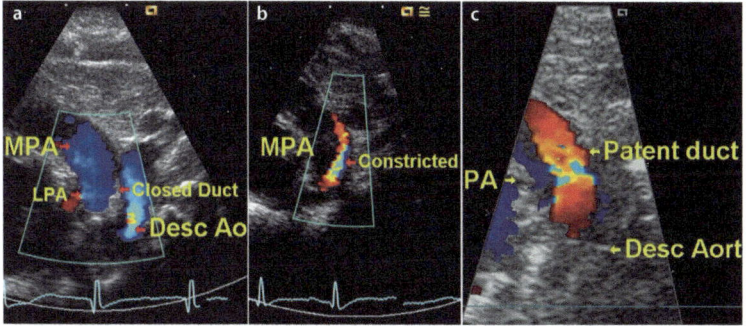

◘ **Fig. 3.3a–c.** Shows varying degrees of ductal constriction as seen with colour Doppler, from (**a**) where the duct is closed with no shunt apparent to (**b**) where the duct is well constricted with a thin shunt stream to (**c**) where the duct is widely patent

optimisation of colour Doppler gain and the velocity scale to minimise colour artefact at the edge of shunt stream map. The diameter of the site of maximum constriction is then measured using the clearest frame in a stored clip [7].

What is the Direction and Velocity of the Shunt?

The direction and velocity of the shunt through the patent duct is a direct product of the relative pressures at each end of the duct. Ductal shunts are complicated because the pressure waves at each end are not synchronous. The pressure wave from the right heart arrives at the duct slightly earlier than the left, partly because of earlier depolarisation but mainly due to proximity to the heart. When the pulmonary pressures are clearly lower than systemic or clearly higher, then the shunt will be respectively left to right or right to left. But as the pulmonary pressures approach systemic, there will be some right to left shunting in early systole well before pulmonary pressures exceed systemic. As pulmonary pressures rise further, the velocity and duration of the right to left shunt will increase (Fig. 3.4).

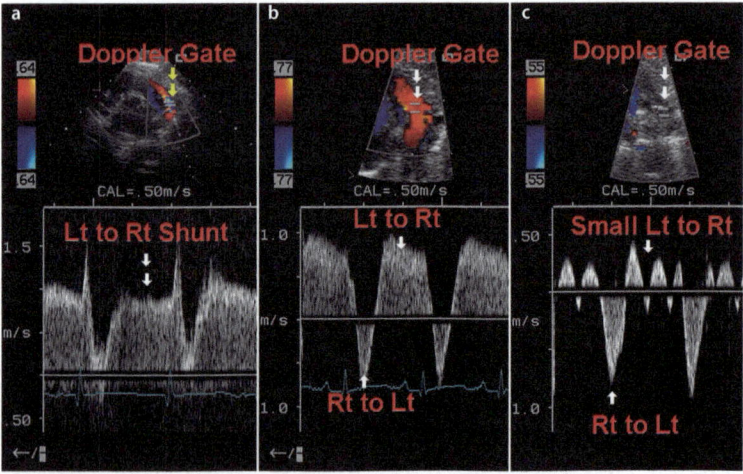

 Fig. 3.4a–c. Shows the range of ductal shunt pattern from pulsatile left to right (**a**) to bidirectional (**b**) to predominantly right to left (**c**)

What is the Hemodynamic Significance of the PDA?

In simple terms this means how much blood is flowing through the ductus. Doppler ultrasound assessments of this are divided into direct and indirect assessments of this flow volume.

The direct assessments are derived from the laws of fluid dynamics, which dictate that flow must be the product of the size (or cross-sectional area) of the vessel and the pressure gradient across that vessel. The size can be estimated as described above from direct 2D imaging together with colour Doppler and the pressure gradient can be estimated from the Doppler velocities. In theory this should allow direct measurement of flow volume in the same way that cardiac output can be measured using the formula:

Stroke Volume = velocity time integral x cross-sectional area (Πr^2)

There are differences here though that will limit the accuracy of such a measure within the ductus. Firstly one cannot assume that the orifice is round, hence the relationship between diameter and cross sectional area will not hold. Secondly the Doppler flow measurements assume laminar flow. This may not be the case for ductal shunting which is often highly turbulent. So while we would not commonly combine these assessments mathematically into a blood flow measure, the physical size (measured as diameter) of the ductus using 2D imaging and/or colour Doppler and the Doppler pattern and velocity of the shunt are commonly used as direct assessment of the significance of the ductal shunt.

The indirect assessments reflect the impact of a left to right shunt on Doppler flow patterns either side of the duct and cardiac chamber dilatation. Blood shunting left to right through the duct will bypass the right heart, increase pulmonary blood flow and so increase the volume load on the left heart. The result is an increase in left atrial diameter, measured as the left atrial to aortic root ratio, increase in left ventricular size, usually measured by end diastolic diameter and increase in left ventricular output (◘ Fig. 3.5).

The other slightly less indirect consequence of a left to right ductal shunt is the disturbance to flow pattern in the major vessels either side of the duct. Blood shunts through the ductus throughout the cardiac cycle with usually more blood moving in systole than diastole. However, because in both circulations, least blood is moving in diastole, more disturbance in flow pattern is seen in diastole than systole. So with increasing ductal shunt size, the normal low velocity antegrade diastolic flow in the post-ductal descending aorta be-

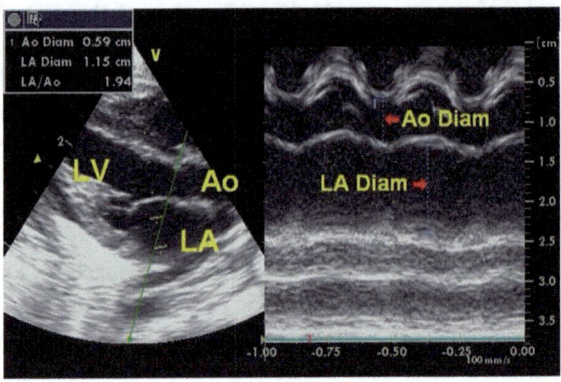

Fig. 3.5. Shows the measurement of the left atrial to aortic root ratio with m-mode. The green line shows the path of the m-mode beam on the 2D image. This LA:Ao at 1.94 is raised

comes progressively absent and then retrograde (**●** Fig. 3.6b). The corollary to this on the other side of the shunt is that the normal low velocity diastolic flow in the left pulmonary artery increases in velocity, indeed all measures of LPA velocity increases including mean velocity (**●** Fig. 3.6a).

The validation of any of these measured runs into the problem of what should be the gold standard. Convention in cardiology is that size of left to right shunts are expressed as a ratio of the pulmonary blood flow (Qp) to the systemic blood flow (Qs), usually written as Qp:Qs. In the paradigm of an isolated ductal shunt, the Qp is represented by the left ventricular output, while the Qs is represented by the right ventricular output. As we can measure both these in the newborn we should be able to measure Qp:Qs. The problem is the common co-existence of a left to right atrial shunt through the foramen ovale. These shunts are variable but can be quite large. We explored the validation of the above direct and indirect measures by measuring Qp:Qs in 69 studies on a group of 24 preterm babies (<1500 g) with a PDA and a small atrial shunts during the first week of life [7]. In this study, Qp:Qs was correlated with PDA diameter, LA:Ao, LV stroke volume and LV output. All these measures had a significant correlation with Qp:Qs but PDA colour Doppler diameter had a much stronger correlation (r=0.8) than LA:Ao (r=0.45), LV stroke volume (r=0.38) or LV output (r=0.43). A diameter above 2 mm was usually associated with a Qp:Qs over 1.7. The velocity of the left to right shunt

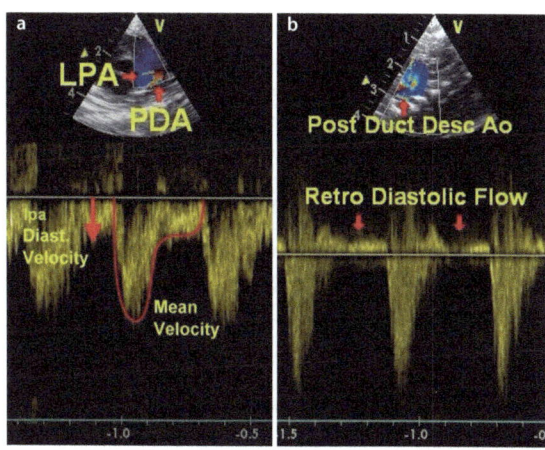

Fig. 3.6a,b. Shows the disturbance of flow either side of a large ductus in (**a**) the left pulmonary artery showing the measurement of peak diastolic velocity and mean velocity. **b** Retrograde diastolic flow in the descending aorta

did not add to these predictive relationships. While this is counter-intuitive, these studies were done in the first week when shunt velocities fall into a narrow range, usually less than 2 m/sec. It is likely that shunt velocity would be a more important determinant of shunt size as they increase after this time. The pattern of diastolic flow in the descending aorta was also compared to Qp:Qs and also showed a significant relationship. With antegrade diastolic flow, the mean Qp:Qs was 1.01; with absent diastolic flow, the mean Qp:Qs was 1.3 and with retrograde diastolic flow, the mean Qp:Qs was 1.7. El Hajjar et al. [8] performed a similar validation but used superior vena cava (SVC) flow as a surrogate for Qs to avoid the confounder of the atrial shunt. They found that ductal diameter over 1.4 mm/kg, LA:Ao over 1.4, LPA mean velocity over 0.42 m/sec or LPA diastolic velocity over 0.2 m/sec, all predicted an LVO:SVC ratio >4 (approx Qp:Qs >2) with more than 90% specificity and sensitivity.

My personal practice is to focus on the direct measures of ductal size and shunt pattern and then use the Doppler flow patterns in the LPA and descending aorta as back up confirmatory measures. In general terms, in a baby born before 30 weeks with a predominantly left to right shunt, ductal diameters less than 1.5 mm will usually not have significant shunts, between 1.5 and 2 mm will be variable and over 2 mm will usually be significant. All ultrasound measures have limitations to accuracy when used in isolation so I usually build up the picture from the patterns of flow in the LPA and descending aorta.

All human injury is defined by the combination of insult and individual host vulnerability. The above only allows you to estimate how much blood is passing through the duct (e.g the insult), it does not allow you to define how important that shunt is to that individual baby (e.g. the vulnerability). Vulnerability is complex but in broad terms the possible injury from a left to right ductal shunt relates to the overload of the pulmonary circulation and the drainage of blood from the systemic circulation.

Impact of the Ductal Shunt on the Lungs

The insult here is the increase in pulmonary blood flow (PBF), this is essentially a passive process resulting from the size of the duct and the pressure gradient as discussed above. The only other limiting factor is the pulmonary vascular resistance, which in turn is one of the determinants of the pressure gradient. The traditional view that pulmonary vascular resistance limits the early hemodynamic impact of the shunt is not born out by studies in the current era. True primary pulmonary hypertension is rare in the preterm infant and even in the early postnatal hours, the dominant direction of shunting is left to right. Large pulmonary blood flows can result when the ductal constriction fails.

Echocardiographic measures of PBF are made complicated by the intracardiac shunts. With an isolated ductal shunt, the LV output will represent pulmonary blood flow but it is unusual that a large ductal shunt is isolated in a preterm baby. This is because the volume load on the left atrium increases pressure and this and the dilatation will drive any shunt through the foramen ovale. These foraminal shunts can be large and on occasions be greater in volume than the ductal shunt [7]. Both these shunts combine to increase PBF, sometimes to a remarkable degree. Qualitatively, these high PBFs can be seen with the ease with which the pulmonary veins flows can be seen on colour Doppler from the subcostal or apical windows. Quantitively, the only way to get an estimate of PBF is to measure the velocities in the root of the left pulmonary artery. Normal values for this have been derived in term babies where mean LPA velocities were usually above 0.2 m/sec [9]. The study of El_Hajjar et al. [8] suggested mean LPA velocity of >0.43 m/sec suggests a large ductal shunt. The problem with this measure is that it is a common in all babies to find acceleration of blood into the LPA, indeed this is a common cause of innocent flow murmurs in all babies but particularly in the preterm baby. The cause of this physiological narrowing at the root of the LPA is not known but it is hypothesised that it may be a consequence of the proximity of the LPA to the ductus, so the LPA can be slightly "gathered up" as the ductus constricts. Experientially I would suggest that narrowing at the root of the LPA is uncommon when the duct is still widely patent. Whatever, LPA mean velocities should be interpreted with this potential confounder in mind.

The clinical impact of high pulmonary blood flow on the lungs is much harder to determine in an individual case. It is suggested from animal models that this high PBF results in higher ventilator requirements but studies of early treatment with indomethacin have shown the reverse of this [10, 11]. It is speculated that this may be due to negative effects on the lungs from indomethacin's impact on fluid balance. For longer-term pulmonary effects, PDA is consistently associated with CLD but again early prophylactic treatment does not reduce CLD rates [12]. This could again be the result of a balance of positive and negative effects of the treatment but currently the data does not support a causative role for the duct in most acute or CLD. The acute pulmonary effect where there is more convincing evidence for a causative role for a ductal shunt is pulmonary haemorrhage. This is actually not blood but hemorrhagic edema. We described 12 babies who developed PH from a cohort of 126 babies born before 30 weeks [2]. At echocardiography close to the time of the PH (pulmonary haemorrhage), these babies had significantly larger ducts (2 mm vs. 0.5 mm) and significantly higher estimated PBF (328 vs. 236 ml/kg/min) than the rest of the cohort. The mean age at time of PH was 38 h with a range from 14 to 55 h, so this seems to be a consequence of early ductal shunting emphasising how the early impact of ductal shunting may be much more important than conventional thinking dictates. In support of this, pulmonary hemorrhage is one of the short-term outcomes reduced by prophylactic indomethacin, particularly when the more minor (probably traumatic) hemorrhage is removed from the analysis [13, 14]. Pulmonary hemorrhage is an acute phenomenon that is difficult to predict from clinical criteria but immaturity and lack of antenatal steroids seem to be risk factors. It is also predicted by early postnatal constriction of the duct. This will be discussed in more detail below. The fact that it occurs in a minority of babies highlights the issue of varying vulnerability in that an insult that is tolerated by many babies is not tolerated by a few. Identifying those few is the challenge in terms of devising therapeutic strategies for the duct.

Impact of the Ductal Shunt on the Systemic Circulation

A left to right ductal shunt drains blood from the systemic circulation, it does this throughout the cardiac cycle, the term "diastolic steal" is one of the great misnomers in neonatology. While the amount drained is passive, the cardiac compensation for the drainage is not and depends on the ability of the left ventricle to increase its output. It does this more through increases in LV stroke volume than heart rate. In this paradigm, the LV output is the sum of the ductal shunt and the systemic blood flow (SBF) and as long as the LV output increases enough to maintain the SBF component, the organs of the body should not suffer. This is complex and ultrasound approaches to this depends on your bias as to whether central or peripheral measures of blood flow are more important.

For all the reasons discussed above, the intracardiac shunts of the transitional circulation confound central measures of SBF. RV output is better at measuring SBF than LV output mainly because PFO shunts are usually (not always) smaller than ductal, but both can be confounded. SVC flow measurement allows a central measure that is not confounded by these shunts and represents the portion of SBF that includes the cerebral blood flow, always the major concern in preterm neonatology. Serial echocardiographic studies have shown that 20 to 30% of babies born before 30 weeks develop very low systemic blood flow usually within the first 12 h [15]. This low SBF state is significantly associated with a range of adverse clinical outcomes. While immaturity is the dominant risk factor, size of the patent ductus was independently related to low SBF but only in the very early scans (at a mean of 5 h). After this time, ductal size was no longer an independent determinant of SBF. Groves et al. [16] also showed a univariant relationship between duct size and low SBF, but in this study it was not significant after controlling for confounding variables, mainly gestation. Within our study, PDA was treated on the basis of usual clinical criteria and we studies SBF at the time of clinical diagnosis and treatment in 27 babies who were at a mean age of 64 h. Mean SVC flow was 74 mls/kg/min (NR 40 to 110) and mean RV output was 242 mls/kg/min (NR

150 to 300) (unpublished observations). While most babies were maintaining SBF, not all were. Two babies had both SVC flow and RV output well below the normal range. These babies were very immature and again this highlights how individual vulnerability can be masked by population summary statistics. These data were derived mainly in the first 2 to 3 postnatal days and there is less systematic study of total SBF in the context of later or prolonged ductal shunting. There is more study of peripheral artery Doppler and flows in the later period and the literature is consistent that if you compare organ blood flows in babies with and without a significant PDA, then the blood flows will be, on average, lower in the babies with PDA. This is true of cerebral blood flow measured by Doppler or NIRS [17] but there is also evidence that the ductal impact on the systemic blood flow may be greater in the post-ductal regions (e.g mesenteric or renal) than the preductal region (e.g cerebral) [18, 19]. Again this is based largely on summary statistics and, with any of these systemic or organ blood flow parameters, we do not have good ways of defining what is pathological in an individual infant. For example, with peripheral artery Doppler measurements the dominant effect of the large PDA shunt is the reduction and eventually reversal of diastolic velocities. This is often quantified by the resistance index (RI); systolic velocity – diastolic velocity/systolic velocity or pulsatility index (PI), which is the same formula as RI except the denominator is mean velocity. The main thing these measures reflect is flow pattern and they are not the same as flow volume although some clinicians use them as such. All peripheral Doppler flow measures are limited by small vessels where it is hard to measure size but fluid dynamics would dictate that mean velocity is likely to be a better measure of flow than velocity pattern. In a study comparing cerebral artery PI and RI with SVC flow, we could find no relationship between these peripheral Doppler measures and the central flow measure. The dominant association of the cerebral artery RI was the size of the ductus arteriosus [20]. So these measures seem to relate to ductal size but there is no good evidence of how we should be using these peripheral arterial Doppler measures in the assessment of the impact on the blood flows in the systemic circulation.

Overall the highest risk period for global reductions in SBF is the first 12 hours after birth. This time seems to be when the ductal shunt has the greatest effects on systemic blood flow possibly because of a limited compensatory ability of the heart in transition. After this transitional period, babies with PDA seem to have lower organ blood flow than those without, particularly in the post ductal regions but most will still be within normal ranges. We still do not know how to define when this becomes pathological in an individual baby.

Prediction of Spontaneous and Therapeutic Ductal Closure

The other, and perhaps not so well recognised, use of echocardiography is to predict closure. The main action of the ductus arteriosus is the powerful smooth muscle induced constriction of the vessel wall. In the term infant, this constriction occurs quickly after birth in almost all babies. In preterm infants, this early postnatal constriction is much more variable. ◘ Figure 3.7 shows the diameter of the ductus at an average of 5 h of age in a cohort of 126 babies born before 30 weeks [2]. The range of constriction at all gestations is apparent. In this study, PDA was treated by usual clinical criteria, e.g development of physical signs and symptoms, usually respiratory. The filled in data points in ◘ Fig. 3.7 shows the babies who were eventually treated for clinically apparent

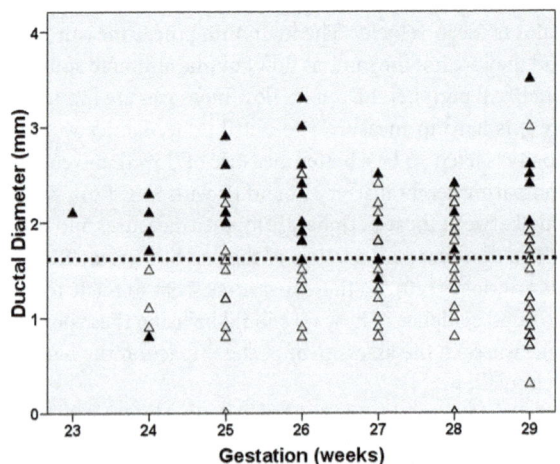

◘ **Fig. 3.7.** Shows the range of ductal constriction at 5 h of age for each gestation in a cohort of 126 babies born before 30 weeks. The dotted line represents the median and the filled in triangles represent babies who later developed a clinically apparent PDA

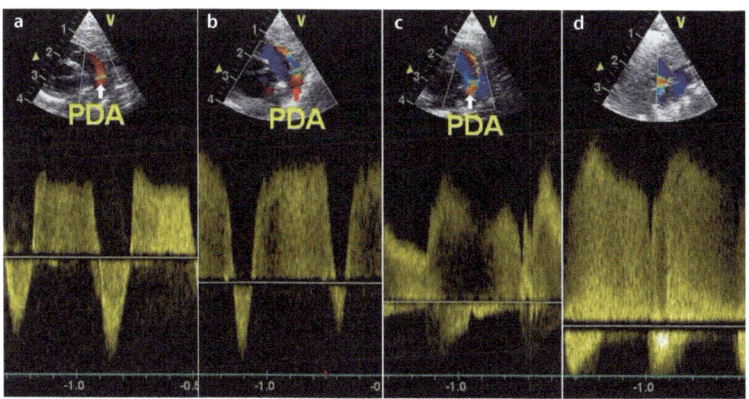

Fig. 3.8a–d. Shows the four shunt flow patterns as described by Su et al. [24]; from pulmonary hypertension (**a**) to growing (**b**) to pulsatile (**c**) to closing (**d**)

PDA. It can be seen that almost all those eventually treated were above the median diameter at 5 h of age, in other words, had below average postnatal constriction. There were exceptions, some, mainly more mature babies had poor postnatal constriction but did close spontaneously and a few mainly less mature, constricted well but then failed to close. Other studies of ductal diameter between 12 and 48 h of age show a similar predictive relationship with eventual treatment [21, 22]. Su et al. [23] described longitudinal assessment of ductal flow pattern to predict development of clinical significance. They described 4 main patterns through which babies tended to evolve as shown in ■ Fig. 3.8; pulmonary hypertension, growing, pulsatile and closing. Babies whose ducts closed tended to go straight from pulmonary hypertension to closing whereas those that became significant progressed to growing pattern and, most specifically, pulsatile pattern. Su et al. did not correlate these patterns with ductal size, we have explored this retrospectively in our data and found a progressive reduction in diameter with the four flow patterns [24]. It may well be that these are two ways of measuring the same thing and as such may be useful as a cross check against each other.

Speed of constriction can also be used to predict response to therapy. Indomethacin produces a rapid constrictive response that is measurable even 2 h after infusion (■ Fig. 3.9) [25]. Mean diameter reduced from 2.4 mm (± 0.6) to 1.6 mm (± 0.6) two hours after the first dose of indomethacin but, as can be

3

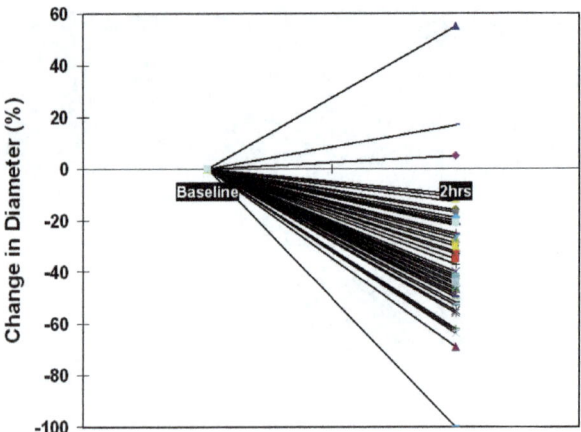

□ Fig. 3.9. Shows the variation in ductal constriction seen two hours after the first dose of early-targeted indomethacin

seen on this graph, there is a wide variation in individual early responsiveness to indomethacin. Experientially we have noted that better early responsiveness predicted closure, so we designed a small trial to test whether this could be used to individualise (and so minimise) the number of indomethacin doses [26]. Babies treated for PDA were randomised to receive either a full course of 3 doses or to have the number of doses tailored to the constrictive response assessed with echo just prior to the second dose. In the echo tailored arm, babies with a good response (diameter less than 1.5 mm) received no more doses where as those with a poor response got all three doses. The closure rates in the two arms were very similar while the echo tailored arm received significantly less indomethacin (median 1 dose vs. 3 doses).

Prediction of spontaneous closure may allow earlier targeted treatment and prediction of therapeutic closure may allow use to minimise dosage of that therapy and so allow minimisation of side effects.

Summary

The current uncertainty in relation to treatment of PDA reflects limitations to our understanding of the pathophysiology of ductal shunting, most particularly which ducts matter to which babies and when they matter. Doppler ultrasound offers a powerful tool with which to assess ductal patency and shunt significance and to allow prediction of spontaneous and therapeutic closure. There is still much to understand about how we can use this tool to understand an individual baby's vulnerability to a ductal shunt and so, when we should treat and when we should leave it alone.

References

1. Evans NJ, Kluckow M (1996) Early significant ductal shunting and intraventricular haemorrhage in ventilated preterm infants. Arch Dis Childhood 75: F183–F186
2. Kluckow M, Evans NJ (2000) High pulmonary blood flow, the duct and pulmonary haemorrhage. J Pediatrics 137: 68–72
3. Noori S, McCoy M, Friedlich P, Bright B, Gottipati V, Seri I, Sekar K (2009) Failure of ductus arteriosus closure is associated with increased mortality in preterm infants. Pediatrics 123: e138–144
4. Benitz WE (2010) Treatment of persistent patent ductus arteriosus in preterm infants: time to accept the null hypothesis? J Perinatol 30: 241–252
5. Bose CL, Laughon MM (2007) Patent ductus arteriosus: lack of evidence for common treatments. Arch Dis Childhood Fetal Neonatal Edition 92: F498–502
6. Laughon MM, Simmons MA, Bose CL (2004) Patency of the ductus arteriosus in the premature infant: is it pathologic? Should it be treated? Curr Opin Pediatrics 16: 146–151
7. Evans NJ, Iyer P (1994) Assessment of ductus arteriosus shunting in preterm infants requiring ventilation: Effect of inter-atrial shunting. J Pediatr 125: 778–785
8. El Hajjar M, Vaksmann G, Rakza T, Kongolo G, Storme L (2005) Severity of the ductal shunt: a comparison of different markers. Arch Dis Child Fetal & Neonatal Edition 90: F419–422
9. Gournay V, Cambonie G, Rozé JC (1998) Doppler echocardiographic assessment of pulmonary blood flow in healthy newborns. Acta Paediatrica 87: 419–423
10. Van Overmeire B, Van de Broek H, Van Laer P, Weyler J, Vanhaesebrouck P (2001) Early versus late indomethacin treatment for patent ductus arteriosus in premature infants with respiratory distress syndrome. J Pediatr 138: 205–211
11. Schmidt B, Roberts R, Fanaroff A et al. (2006) Indomethacin prophylaxis, patent ductus arteriosus and the risk of bronchopulmonary dysplasia: Further analyses from the Trial of Indomethacin Prophylaxis in Preterms. J Pediatr 148: 730–734
12. Fowlie PW, Davis PG, McGuire W (2010) Prophylactic intravenous indomethacin for preventing mortality and morbidity in preterm infants. Cochrane Database of Systematic Reviews, Issue 7: CD000174
13. Schmidt B, Davis P, Moddemann D, Ohlsson A, Roberts RS, Saigal S, Solimano A, Vincer M, Wright LL (2001) Trial of Indomethacin Prophylaxis in Preterms Investigators. Long-term effects of indomethacin prophylaxis in extremely-low-birth-weight infants. N Eng J Med 344: 1966–1972

14. Alfaleh K, Smyth JA, Roberts RS, Solimano A, Asztalos EV, Schmidt B (2008) Trial of Indomethacin Prophylaxis in Preterms Investigators. Prevention and 18-month outcomes of serious pulmonary hemorrhage in extremely low birth weight infants: results from the trial of indomethacin prophylaxis in preterms. Pediatrics 121: e233–238

15. Kluckow M, Evans NJ (2000) Low superior vena cava flow and intraventricular haemorrhage in preterm infants. Arch Dis Child 82: F188–194

16. Groves AM, Kuschel CA, Knight DB, Skinner JR (2008) Does retrograde diastolic flow in the descending aorta signify impaired systemic perfusion in preterm infants? Pediatric Res 63: 89–94

17. Lemmers PM, Toet MC, van Bel F (2008) Impact of patent ductus arteriosus and subsequent therapy with indomethacin on cerebral oxygenation in preterm infants. Pediatrics 121: 142–147

18. El-Khuffash A, Higgins M, Walsh K, Molloy EJ (2008) Quantitative assessment of the degree of ductal steal using celiac artery blood flow to left ventricular output ratio in preterm infants. Neonatology 93: 206–212

19. Groves AM, Kuschel CA, Knight DB, Skinner JR (2008) Does retrograde diastolic flow in the descending aorta signify impaired systemic perfusion in preterm infants? Pediatric Res 63: 89–94

20. Evans N, Kluckow M, Simmons M, Osborn D (2002) Which to measure, systemic or organ blood flow? Middle cerebral artery and superior vena cava flow in preterm infants. Arch Dis Child 87: F181–F184

21. Kwinta P, Rudzinski A, Kruczek P, Kordon Z, Pietrzyk JJ (2009) Can early echocardiographic findings predict patent ductus arteriosus? Neonatology 95: 141–148

22. Kluckow M, Evans NJ (1995) Early echocardiographic prediction of symptomatic patent ductus arteriosus in preterm infants requiring mechanical ventilation. J Pediatrics 127: 774–779

23. Su BH, Watanabe T, Shimizu M, Yanagisawa M (1997) Echocardiographic assessment of patent ductus arteriosus shunt flow pattern in premature infants. Arch Dis Child Fetal Neonatal 77: F36–F40

24. Condò M, Evans N, Bellù R, Kluckow M (2011) Echocardiographic assessment of ductal significance: retrospective comparison of two methods. Arch Dis Child (submitted for publication)

25. Osborn DA, Kluckow M, Evans N (2003) Effect of early targeted indomethacin on the ductus arteriosus and blood flow to the upper body and brain in the preterm infant. Arch Dis Child 88: F477–F482

26. Browning-Carmo K, Evans N, Paradisis M (2009) Duration of indomethacin treatment of the preterm patent ductus arteriosus as directed by echocardiography. J Pediatrics 155: 819–822

Evaluation of the Open Duct Using Systolic Time Intervals and Doppler Sonography of Peripheral Arteries

E. Robel-Tillig

There have been a lot of studies on the assessment of ductal shunting during the last decades. While neonatologists and pediatric cardiologists discuss advantages and limitations of different echocardiographical measures to assess whether an open duct requires treatment, echocardiography should never replace the overall clinical evaluation, but add to it.

The focus of this chapter is on the assessment of the patent duct using left ventricular systolic time intervals and flow patterns in peripheral arteries.

Systolic Time Intervals

The first studies describing the evaluation of systolic time intervals for the assessment of the hemodynamic situation in fetuses and neonates were published in the late 1980s by perinatologists and neonatologists. These investigations aimed to define normal values for left and right ventricular systolic time intervals in fetuses and neonates. Some publications reported changes of these parameters in fetuses after premature rupture of membranes or compared the time intervals in neonates after spontaneous vaginal delivery or after cesarean section. In neonates with congenital heart disease, particularly in lesions with intracardiac shunts impacting on hemodynamics, systolic time intervals are difficult to interpret. In neonatology, however, where most infants have a structurally normal heart, systolic time intervals may be of utmost interest to assess the hemodynamic effects of the open duct, particularly because systolic time intervals can be measured non-invasively, and quite easily and quickly by Doppler ultrasound, and consequently the infant is hardly disturbed or stressed by the examination.

Definitions of the Ejection Time and the Pre-Ejection Period

We measure left and right ventricular ejection time and left and right ventricular pre-ejection period.

The ejection time is measured as the time interval from the opening of the aortic or the pulmonary valve until the closure of the aortic or the pulmonary valve, respectively. The ejection times correlate strongly with the left or the right ventricular stroke volume and hence cardiac output.

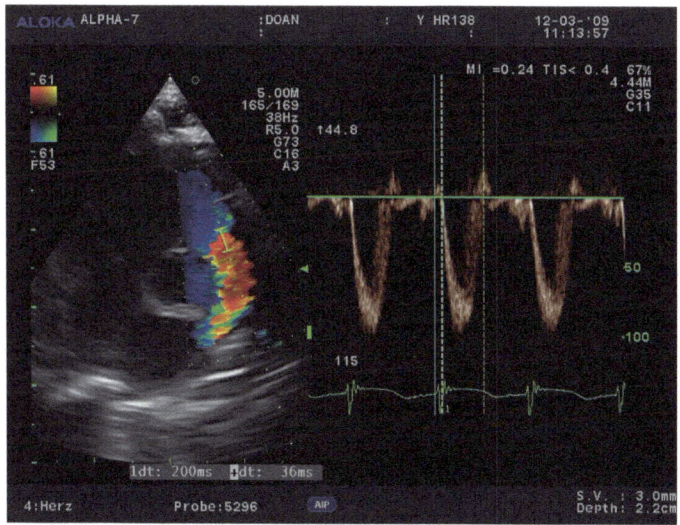

Fig. 4.1. Assessment of left ventricular systolic time intervals by Doppler sonography

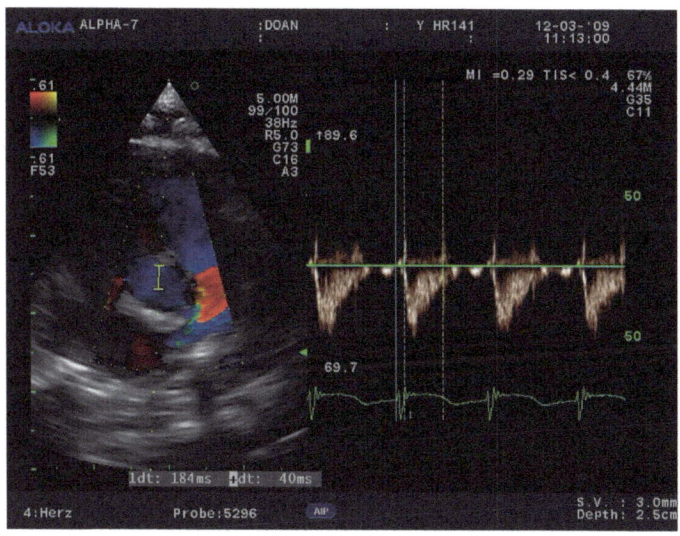

Fig. 4.2. Assessment of right ventricular time intervals by Doppler sonography

The pre-ejection period is the short isovolumetric contraction phase of the myocardium and depends on both, myocardial contractility and afterload. It is measured as the time between the first deflection (usually the onset of the Q-wave) of the concomitantly displayed ECG on the screen of the ultrasound device and the Doppler signal indicating the opening of the aortic or the pulmonary valve (◘ Figs. 4.1 and 4.2).

How to Measure the Ejection Time and the Pre-Ejection Period?

It is important to perform the measurements in an environment that keeps the neonate comfortable. Cold babies may cry and struggle, unnecessarily hindering the examination and rendering the retrievable hemodynamic information less meaningful.

The infant must be examined in a supine position. The ultrasound machine needs to be configured appropriately for neonates with an integrated ECG recording.

To examine the neonatal heart, three standard planes are used. These planes or axes correspond to the mathematical x, y, and z- axes and are at a right angle to each other. These planes are called the long parasternal axis, the short parasternal axis and the four-chamber view. To measure systolic time intervals the short parasternal axis should be used. Short parasternal axis views are obtained from the parasternal position by rotating the transducer 90° from the long parasternal axis. The left and the right atrium, the tricuspid valve, and the right ventricular outflow tract can be visualized around the centrally positioned aortic valve and the origins of the coronary arteries. By tilting up towards the sternal notch a higher cut demonstrates the right ventricular outflow tract, pulmonary arteries and the patent duct.

For the measurement of left ventricular time intervals the sample volume can be placed in the aortic valve and for right ventricular time intervals in the pulmonary valve, respectively.

Reference Ranges for the Ejection Time and the Pre-Ejection Period

Several study groups determined reference ranges for the systolic time intervals as measured by Doppler sonography. Whereas the left ventricular pre-ejection period (LPEP) does not change with gestational age in neonates, the ejection time (LVET) is shorter in preterm infants than in term infants. Whereas the LPEP increases, the LVET decreases in both groups on day five of life compared with the first day of life. Consequently, the ratio of LPEP/ LVET is rising from day one to day five (■ Table 4.1).

The timing and duration of right ventricular time intervals change with changes of pulmonary arterial pressure. Right ventricular pre-ejection period is directly related to the pulmonary arterial pressure. As the pulmonary arterial pressure increases, the ratio of RPEP/ RVET rises.

Because the effects of a patent ductus arteriosus on right ventricular time intervals are less predictable, we will concentrate on left ventricular time intervals in neonates with persistent duct.

Left ventricular ejection time correlates negatively with heart rate. However, if the heart rate is between 135 bpm and 160 bpm the correlation is not significant and a time correction is not necessary.

Hemodynamic changes associated with a patent duct's predominant left-to-right shunt are reflected in predictable changes in left ventricular systolic time intervals in neonates. In infants with a PDA with left to right shunt, the left ventricular pre-ejection period is shorter (<0.35 ms), and the left ventricular ejection time is prolonged as a result of an increased left ventricular stroke volume/cardiac output. Consequently, the ratio of LPEP/ LVET is decreased (<0.32).

■ **Table 4.1.** Reference ranges for left ventricular ejection time (LVET) and left ventricular pre-ejection period (LPEP)

	First day of life	Fifth day of life
LVET (preterm neonates)	155–172 ms	148–165 ms
LVET (term neonates)	174–198 ms	168–188 ms
LPEP (preterms and terms)	35–55 ms	40–58 ms
Ratio LPEP/LVET	0.33–0.42	0.35–0.44

It is necessary to appreciate that other pathophysiological changes in neonatal hemodynamics may also influence systolic time intervals. As we mentioned, a high heart rate, frequently encountered in neonates with a significant PDA, decreases the LVET. A shortening of LVET is also seen in infants with severe hypovolemia. In contrast, if the myocardial contractility is poor, e.g., secondary to a long-standing volume overload due to PDA, the LVET will be prolonged. The LPEP, normally reduced in neonates with a persistent duct, can also be prolonged due to a reduced myocardial contractility in a severely ill baby. Therefore it is important to take further parameters into consideration to define a significant PDA and to deduce an indication for therapy.

Doppler Sonographic Blood Flow Parameters of Peripheral Arteries

Circulatory effects of patent ductus arteriosus do not only affect left ventricular output and left ventricular systolic time intervals but also cause changes in end-organ blood flow. Important left-to-right shunt through a large PDA can cause ductal steal and consequently abnormal flow patterns with high pulsatility indices in the descending aorta, and the cerebral, intestinal, and renal arteries. It is necessary to measure systolic, diastolic, and mean blood flow velocities, and resistance and pulsatility indices in these vessels to evaluate the degree of the blood flow disturbance associated with the patent duct.

Measurement of Blood Flow Parameters of Peripheral Arteries

Descending Aorta

Diastolic aortic pressure is low with a large left-to-right ductal shunt owing to ductal steal. Blood passing down the descending aorta during systole goes back upwards through the arterial duct and into the pulmonary arteries during diastole. The direction of blood flow in the descending aorta can be easily assessed from a transabdominal view of the descending aorta distally of the duct. The results of qualitative assessment of flow direction are not modified by an angled insonation. However, air in the abdomen of the preterm infant could be a problem. Diastolic retrograde or absent flow in the descending aorta is associated with an increased cardiac output. There is also a strong correlation with a decreased flow volume in the descending aorta. A ductal diameter greater than the median of normative data for the gestational age, is associated with a disturbed blood flow in the descending aorta. In conclusion, a large duct with predominant left to right shunting and increased left ventricular output may be predicted if absent or retrograde diastolic flow is observed in the descending aorta. Infants with a high volume ductal shunt may have preserved upper body but reduced lower body perfusion.

Anterior Cerebral Artery

Measurement of blood-flow parameters in the anterior cerebral artery is commonly used in neonatal clinical practice. It is easy to perform through the anterior fontanelle. In infants with a large patent duct we can observe a ductal steal resulting in an absent or even retrograde diastolic flow (■ Fig. 4.3). The pulsatility index is high. However, it is important to appreciate that similar Doppler findings are also seen in neonates with severe brain edema. Therefore, the general clinical condition of the baby has to be taken into account to avoid a misinterpretation of the Doppler results.

Superior Mesenteric Artery

Similar assessments of the effect of ductal steal on peripheral perfusion can be made in the mesenteric artery using a subcostal position of the transducer. In cases with a ductal steal phenomenon, we measure decreased, absent or reversed diastolic flow in the superior mesenteric artery (■ Fig. 4.4).

Again the general condition of the infant must be taken into account to prevent misinterpretation because neonates with intrauterine growth restriction often suffer from severe intestinal blood flow disturbances in the absence of a patent duct. These flow disturbances, also characterized by absent or reversed diastolic blood flow in the intestinal vessels, are frequently seen in growth-restricted infants with clinical intestinal problems such as feeding intolerance, abdominal distension, or delayed meconium excretion.

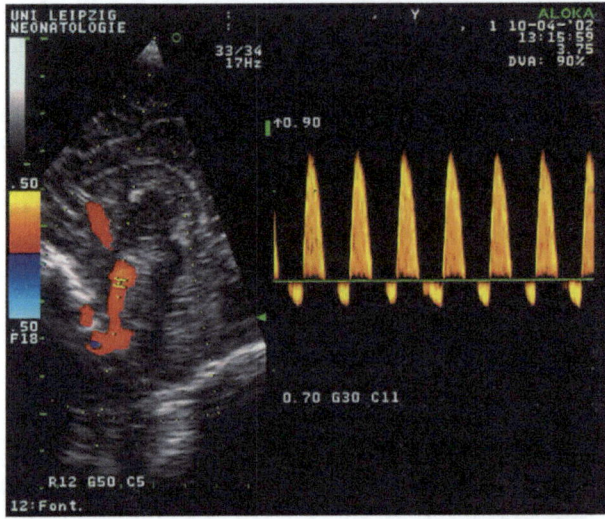

Fig. 4.3. Ductal steal phenomenon in the anterior cerebral artery with diastolic reverse flow

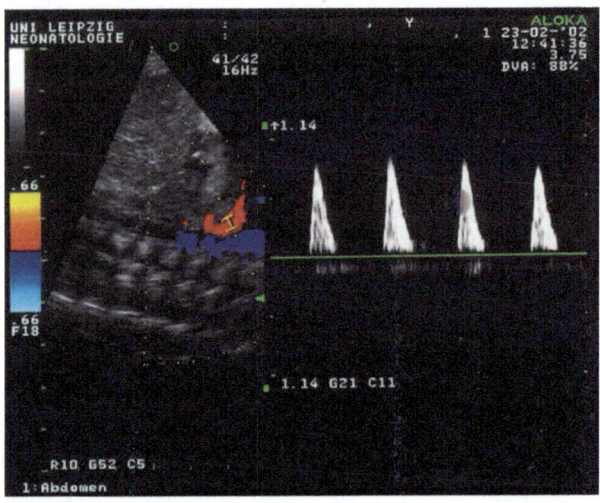

Fig. 4.4. Ductal steal phenomenon in the superior mesenteric artery with absent diastolic flow

Renal Artery

The third type of peripheral vessels which are easily assessed by Doppler sonography and which are also characterized by impaired diastolic flow caused by ductal steal in infants with large left-to-right shunts through an open duct, are the left and right renal arteries.

When interpreting the findings one has once more to appreciate that infants with renal failure, for instance after severe birth asphyxia, or with prenatally disturbed renal function can also demonstrate absent or reversed diastolic blood flow in the renal arteries.

Summary and Conclusion

As described above, left ventricular systolic time intervals in addition to Doppler ultrasound assessment of the blood flow velocities in the peripheral arteries are useful markers for assessment of the hemodynamic changes associated with an open duct and may help to identify infants in whom the patent duct has the most profound circulatory effects. Like other parameters, these measurements are qualitative rather than quantitative and variable data on repeatability have been reported.

Nevertheless, we would advise to add the methods described above to the diagnostic program for assessing the patent duct because the measurements are uncomplicated, quickly performed, and non-invasive.

References

1. Groves AM, Kuschel CA, Knight DR, Skinner DR (2008) Does retrograde diastolic flow in the descending aorta signify impaired systemic perfusion in preterm infants? Pediatr Res 56: 89–94
2. Shimada S, Kasai T, Hoshi A, Murata A, Chida S (2003) Circulatory effects of patent ductus arteriosus in extremely low-birth-weight infants. Pediatrics 45: 255–263
3. Puviani G, Cirelli G, Venezia M, Zanni G (1986) Systolic time intervals in patent ductus arteriosus before and after corrective surgery. Clin Cardiol 16: 818–821
4. Wunderlich M, Koehler J, Rohwedder G, Hubricht R, Müller A (1986) Determination of systolic time intervals of fetal heart as an additional diagnosis sub partu. Zentrbl Gynäkol 24: 1500–1507

5. Kagyia A, Echizeniya N, Hamada A, Tachizzaki T, Satoh S, Siotoh Y (1989) The evaluation of systolic time intervals and impedance cardiogram of neonates. Nippon Sanka Gakkai Zasshi 41: 601–608
6. Ruckhäberle KE, Vogtmann C, Forberg J, Viehweg B, Chiakha S (1989) Fetal systolic time intervals in threatened premature labor and their relation to therapeutic efforts. Z Geburtsh Perinatol 193: 129–133
7. Makihara K, Hata T, Hata K, Kiato M (1993) Echocardiographic assessment of systolic time intervals in vaginal and caesarean delivered neonates. Ann J Perinatol 10: 53–57
8. Hata T, Senoh D, Makihara K, Hatta K, Takamiya O, Kioto M (1989) Fetal cardiac time intervals determined by Doppler echocardiography. J Perinatol Med 17: 85–92
9. Cui W, Robertson DA, Chen Z, Madronero LF, Cuneo BF (2008) Systolic and diastolic time intervals measured from Doppler tissue imaging: normal values and Z- score tables, and effects of age, heart rate, and body surface. J Am Soc Echocardiogr 21: 361–370
10. Robel-Tillig E, Knuepfer M, Pulzer F, Vogtmann C (2003) Dopplers sonographic findings in neonates with persistent ductus arteriosus. Early Hum Dev 83: 307–312
11. Lindner W, Döhlemann C, Schneider K, Versmold H (1985) Heart rate and systolic time intervals in healthy newborn infants: longitudinal study. Pediatr Cardiol 6: 117–121
12. Agata Y, Hirashi S, Hirota J, Hirnigucchi K (1994) Regional blood flow distribution and left ventricular output during early neonatal life: a quantitative ultrasonographic assessment. Pediatr Res 36: 805–810
13. Jin VT, Chiu NC, Hung HY, Chang JH (2005) Cerebral hemodynamic change and intraventricular hemorrhage in very low birth weight infants with patent ductus arteriosus. Ultrasound Med Biol 31: 197–202
14. Freeman- Ladd M, Cohen JB, Carver JD, Hutch JC (2005) The hemodynamic effect of neonatal patent ductus arteriosus shunting on superior mesenteric artery. J Perinatol 25: 459–462

Competitive Inhibition of Bilirubin-Albumin Binding by Ibuprofen

L. Desfrère, C. Huon

Introduction

Hemodynamically significant patent ductus arteriosus (hsPDA) has gained increasing clinical importance on account of the increasing chance of survival of very preterm infants. The incidence of hsPDA varies from 40 to 70% on the third day of life [1]. HsPDA is associated with several co-morbidities like bronchopulmonary dysplasia, intraventricular hemorrhage, necrotizing enterocolitis, and death. Since 1976, inhibition of prostaglandin synthesis with indomethacin has been widely used in the prophylactic or curative treatment of hsPDA. Recently, ibuprofen (IBU) has become increasingly used because of a comparable efficacy in promoting ductal closure, with fewer adverse effects on renal, mesenteric and cerebral blood flows [2, 3]. However, a potential side effect of IBU is the decrease of bilirubin binding capacity of albumin and thereby an increased risk of bilirubin neurotoxicity. In many neonatal intensive care units, hsPDA is preferentially treated in the first week of life, typically at the same time when the bilirubin pool is increased. IBU is intensely bound to albumin (95%) and can displace bilirubin from its albumin binding sites at high concentrations in vitro [4–7]. Conversely, though indomethacin is also firmly bound to albumin, it does not seem to affect the bilirubin binding to albumin [8]. Until recently, IBU remained to be evaluated concerning its potential for displacement of bilirubin from albumin in vivo.

Hyperbilirubinemic Encephalopathy in Preterm Infants

The net accumulation of bilirubin over time, referred to as bilirubin load or miscible bilirubin pool, depends on the bilirubin production rate, excretion rate and enterohepatic recirculation. Neonatal hyperbilirubinemia is a transient state generally considered as benign except when high plasma levels lead to bilirubin encephalopathy or kernicterus. Overall improvements in treatment (phototherapy and exchange transfusion) for hyperbilirubinemia have resulted in a marked decrease in the reports of kernicterus in term infants. However, kernicterus continued to be reported in preterm infants, some at total bilirubin concentrations (TBC) previously considered as safe in the absence of acute neurologic signs [9, 10]. Moreover, an association between peak TBC and death or neurodevelopmental impairment, psychomotor developmental index <70 and hearing impairment has been shown in extremely preterm infants [11]. These reports raise concerns about potential bilirubin neurotoxicity at low TBC in preterm infants and the quantification of this risk is widely discussed. Even though TBC and/or bilirubin-albumin molar ratio (MR) may be used to estimate the risk of bilirubin neurotoxicity in term neonates, they remain unreliable predictors of bilirubin neurotoxicity in preterm infants [12]. Alternative predictors for bilirubin neurotoxicity in premature neonates could therefore improve clinical practice. Experimental and clinical data suggest that the measurement of unbound bilirubin (UB) which can easily cross the blood-brain barrier reflects more reliably the bilirubin load in the brain and might improve the risk assessment of bilirubin neurotoxicity in preterm infants [13]. Elevated UB have been associated with kernicterus in sick preterm infants [14]. Ahlfors et al. reported that abnormal automated auditory brainstem responses were associated with increased UB but not with increased TBC [15]. Indeed, UB may vary widely for a given TBC because the binding capacity of albumin may be decreased by many clinical and physiological variables. Moreover, the bilirubin binding capacity of albumin varies significantly between neonates [16], is impaired in sick neonates [17] and increases with increasing gestational and postnatal age [16, 18]. However, the neurotoxic UB threshold remains debatable although UB concentrations >1.0 µg/dL discriminated toxic levels from asymptomatic preterm neonates with both a high sensitivity and specificity [13]. Finally, the risk of bilirubin neurotoxicity is not simply a function of UB concentration or TBC alone but rather a combination of both (miscible bilirubin pool) as well as the tendency of UB to enter the tissue. In addition, other determinants of the neurotoxic effects of bilirubin are the damage of the blood brain barrier, the duration of exposure and the susceptibility of the cells of the central nervous system to be damaged by bilirubin [19]. It was suggested that UB is a substrate for P-glycoprotein which is pivotal for the energy-dependent cellular efflux of lipophilic substrates [20]. Hanko et al. demonstrated that several drugs (including IBU), known to inhibit P-glycoprotein have a direct effect on the bilirubin levels in the brain [21].

Measurement of Unbound Bilirubin Concentrations

Clinical laboratory measurement of UB is not generally available. The peroxidase method, which is used to measure both TBC and UB, is the most widely used test [22]. However, the instrument and reagents are difficult to obtain and are primarily used for research purposes. The standard peroxidase method, using a 1:42-fold serum dilution, has several limitations to evaluate a bilirubin binding competitor. First, serum dilution has been shown to alter bilirubin-albumin binding. It yields false low UB results in infants with elevated levels of a competing albumin ligand [23]. Furthermore, this method uses a single peroxidase concentration, which underestimates UB, an error that worsens as the actual UB level increases. Ahlfors, recently developed a modified peroxidase method in order to overcome these problems [24]. This method requires small sample volumes (50 µl), minimizes the dilution (2-fold sample dilution) and uses at least 2 concentrations of the enzyme. This modified method provides 5- to 10-fold higher UB values than the standard method. Ahlfors demonstrated that, in vitro, known competing ligands (sulfisoxazole and benzoate) induced a large increase of UB at minimal dilution while their impact on UB concentration was almost negligible when assayed at the 1:42-fold dilution [25].

Bilirubin-Albumin Binding and Bilirubin Displacers

In the circulation, most bilirubin is bound to albumin whereas a relatively small fraction remains unbound. UB can enter in the extravascular (brain) compartments at a rate proportional to the UB level. For a given TBC, the UB concentration is inversely proportional to the albumin concentration and to the bilirubin-albumin association constant (K), a measure of its intrinsic ability to bind albumin. The relation can be expressed by the equation:

UB = TBC-UB/K (A-TBC+UB)

The bilirubin binding to albumin may be affected by the presence of a competitor for albumin binding inducing a decrease of the apparent bilirubin-albumin association constant with a release of UB even at a low MR. Several drugs and preservatives used in these medications have been shown to displace bilirubin from albumin [26]. Sulfisoxazole is the most widely studied drug in relation to clinical [27] and experimental settings [28] of kernicterus. Other substances also have a strong effect on bilirubin-albumin binding like benzoate, sulfamethaxazole, ceftriaxone, cefotetan, carbenicillin, moxalactam,

▣ **Table 5.1.** Bilirubin displacers at therapeutic dosages		
Strong displacers	**Weak displacers**	**No displacing effect**
▬ Benzoate	▬ Ampicillin	▬ Dopamine
▬ Sulfisoxazole	▬ Oxacillin	▬ Dobutamine
▬ Sulfamethaxazole	▬ Aminophylline	▬ Morphine
▬ Ceftriaxone	▬ Nafcillin	▬ Fentanyl
▬ Cefotetan	▬ Phenobarbital	▬ Insulin
▬ Carbenicillin	▬ Phenylbutazone	▬ Indomethacin
▬ Moxalactam	▬ Papaverine	▬ Vitamins
▬ Dicloxacillin	▬ Furosemide	▬ Aminoglycosides
▬ Methicillin	▬ Ibuprofen	▬ Thyroxine
▬ Cefazolin		

dicloxacillin, methicillin and cefazolin. The simultaneous use of these drugs should be avoided as long as there is a risk for bilirubin neurotoxicity. Among the drugs that are commonly used in preterm infants, some are considered weak displacers of bilirubin (▣ Table 5.1). Furthermore, elevated free fatty acid levels have been shown to displace bilirubin from albumin in newborns [29]. IBU also has a significant bilirubin displacing effect, which depends on: the plasma concentrations of albumin and IBU, the albumin association constants for bilirubin and drug and TBC at the time of IBU administration.

IBU Concentrations During Treatment of hsPDA

Aranda et al. first reported high mean IBU concentrations (180 ± 11 μg/mL) in infants receiving prophylactic IBU at the current dose regimen (10–5–5 mg/kg every 24 h) within 3 h postnataly [30]. Such high concentrations have not been reported again in further clinical studies including very early IBU administration within 6 h of birth [31–34]. Most concentrations ranged between 10 and 70 μg/mL. However, high IBU levels (>100 μg/mL) may be reached in rare cases with the current dose regimen because of the marked inter-individual pharmacokinetic variability [30]. Several factors may influence the IBU pharmacokinetics in these sick preterm infants such as the clinical condition (respiratory status with associated acid-base imbalances, fluid shifts after birth, declining albumin levels, and increasing bilirubin levels) and pharmacogenetic factors (expression of the cytochrome P450 complex which metabolizes IBU). Moreover, co-administration of drugs may induce direct drug interactions, alter albumin binding, influence the IBU clearance, or induce hepatic metabolism.

In order to determine the range of observed IBU concentrations during treatment of hsPDA, all individual plasma pharmacokinetic data obtained during the clinical development of IBU (Pedea®, Orphan Europe) were retrospectively pooled. Only clinical data of curative treatment of hsPDA were considered. IBU concentrations were assayed with high-pressure liquid chromatography. Individual plasma concentrations were obtained either directly on racemic IBU (R + S enantiomers) in a double-blind dose-finding study (n=42) [32] or by adding R- and S-IBU concentrations at each time point in 3 other studies. The primary objectives of these latter studies were to determine the risks of pulmonary hypertension in premature infants delivered before 28 weeks gestational age (n=14) [35], to compare the incidence of surgical ligation of hsPDA after prophylactic versus curative IBU treatment (n=10) [36] and to study bilirubin displacement during IBU treatment in premature infants below 32 weeks gestational age (n=33) [37]. According to the schedules of studies, different pharmacokinetic sampling times were obtained: just before, after and 6 h after the loading dose of IBU, just before and after the second infusion, just before and after the third infusion, 72 h after the start of the infusion of the loading dose of IBU. Two hundred-seventy-nine samples were obtained from the ninety-nine patients enrolled in the 4 studies. Mean (SD) concentrations of IBU at each sampling time after the various dose-regimens are shown in ■ Table 5.2. Seventy-two patients (228 samples) were treated by the currently recommended IBU dose regimen of 10 mg/kg followed by 5 mg/kg/d for two more days. The concentrations were maximal at the end of the infusion of the loading dose in all patients except thirteen with maximum concentrations after the first or second maintenance dose. Concentrations above 100 µg/mL occurred only in 2 patients after the loading dose (■ Fig. 5.1). In the dose-range study, among seventeen patients treated with a dose-regimen of 15–7.5–7.5 mg/kg/d only one patient had a concentration above 100 µg/mL (i.e. 103 µg/mL) after the loading dose. One infant had an accidental overdose at the first infusion (50 mg/kg) with a maximal IBU concentration of 148 µg/mL. Therefore, this retrospective analysis of IBU concentrations over time suggests that concentrations above 100 µg/mL should be rare.

■ Table 5.2. Mean concentrations (SD) of IBU at the different sampling times after curative treatment at various dose-regimens

Dose regimens (mg/kg/d)	Peak post LD (µg/mL)	6 hours post LD (µg/mL)	24 hours post LD (µg/mL)	Peak post MD1 (µg/mL)	48 hours post LD (µg/mL)	Peak post MD2 (µg/mL)	72 hours post LD (µg/mL)
5–2.5–2.5 (n=8)	25.2 (9.3)						21.3 (13.2)
10–5–5 (n=72)	49.6 (21.6)	32.1 (9.8)	24.7 (8.5)	48.9 (12.8)	15.5 (10.2)	40 (14.8)	21.7 (12.5)
15–7.5–7.5 (n=17)	58.1 (15.6)						15.6 (13)
20 (n=1)	68						
50 (n=1)	143						

LD loading dose, MD1 first maintenance dose, MD2 second maintenance dose

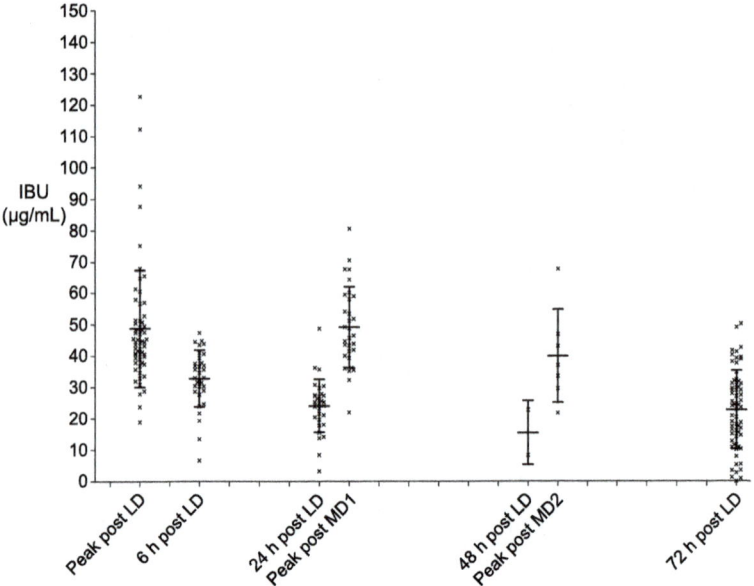

⬛ **Fig. 5.1.** Individual plasma concentrations of IBU during the currently recommended dose regimen of 10 mg/kg followed by 5 mg/kg/d for two more days. The plain line and T-bar represent the mean concentrations and 1 SD observed at the different times, respectively.

Bilirubin-Albumin Displacing Effect of IBU in Vitro

The effects of high concentrations of IBU on bilirubin-albumin binding in newborn serum have been demonstrated in in-vitro studies. However, they have not been equally conclusive. Cooper-Peel et al. first reported the effect of IBU on bilirubin-albumin binding by measuring the reverse displacement effect of bilirubin on the binding of the drug [4]. At an IBU concentration of 750 µmol/l (155 µg/mL) and MR of 0.5, UB was increased by factor 4. The authors concluded that IBU might increase the risk of bilirubin neurotoxicity. These results were confirmed by Ahlfors et al. using the peroxidase-diazo method at a 1.6-fold sample dilution to measure the concentrations of UB in pooled plasma from jaundiced newborn infants [5]. The UB concentrations were significantly increased at an IBU concentration of 100 µg/mL. Neverthe-

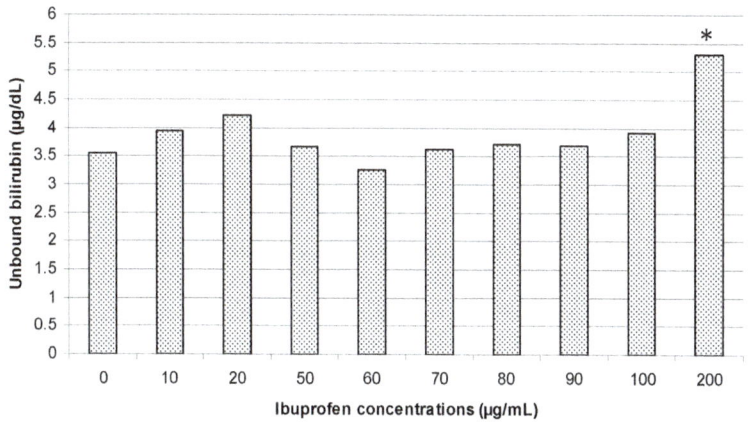

■ Fig. 5.2. Mean UB concentrations in the absence and in the presence of IBU concentrations between 10 and 200 µg/mL. *p<0.001 as compared to control without drug.

less, no increase of UB was shown at concentrations generally observed in clinical practice at the recommended dose regimen (i.e. 50 µg/mL). In another study using the saturation index of Odell and testing different MRs of 0.5, 1, 1.5 and 2 with bilirubin concentrations of 5 or 10 mg/dL and IBU concentrations of 142.5, 200 and 285 µg/mL [6], significant displacement of bilirubin from albumin was only observed for the highest MR and the highest concentration of IBU (285 µg/mL). Recently, Soligard et al. confirmed the displacing effect of IBU at a concentration of 177 µg/mL and a dose-related linear relationship between IBU concentrations and bilirubin displacement [7]. All of these in-vitro studies showed a bilirubin-albumin binding displacing effect of IBU at concentrations higher than those generally observed during hsPDA treatment in preterm infants. A recent in-vitro study reassessed the effect of IBU on bilirubin-albumin binding over a range covering the concentrations of IBU that have been observed in the clinical development of Pedea®. Total bilirubin and UB concentrations without IBU and in the presence of raising concentrations of IBU were determined using the peroxidase-diazo method on a pool of excess plasma collected during a clinical study in preterm newborn infants [38]. The mean TBC without IBU was 6.6 mg/dL and the albumin level 2.87 g/dL, leading to a MR of 0.26. No significant effect of IBU was observed on bilirubin-albumin binding at IBU concentrations from 10 to

100 µg/mL, corresponding to those observed in clinical studies. Only at a concentration of 200 µg/mL, IBU significantly increased the unbound bilirubin by 1.5-fold (◻ Fig. 5.2). This later in-vitro study suggests that significant displacement of bilirubin from albumin should be extremely rare in clinical practice at the recommended IBU dose regimen.

Bilirubin-Albumin Displacing Effect of IBU in Vivo

The effect may be different in vivo, and it is more difficult to study the bilirubin-albumin-IBU interaction because of the rapidly changing UB and TBC [5]. A single measurement of UB concentrations after administration of the drug may not provide an accurate evaluation of the potential effect of the drug. In vivo, the increase of UB induced by the reduced bilirubin-albumin affinity is attenuated by the diffusion into tissues which is not the case in vitro [7]. In animal models, the UB concentration after a sharp and transient increase returned to its pre-treatment value despite continued infusion of the displacing drug [8]. TBC should decrease under these conditions. Until now, no trial specifically studying the potential bilirubin-displacing effect of IBU with serial and simultaneous measurements of IBU, TBC and UB during the course of IBU treatment has been published.

In 2 recent studies, IBU was shown to be associated with an increase of TBC in preterm infants with hsPDA [39, 40]. These studies have several limitations. First, UB was not measured and TBC levels are not appropriate to estimate the risk of kernicterus through bilirubin-albumin displacement. Theoretically, if UB was increased (due to displacement by IBU) TBC should decrease. Zecca et al. interestingly hypothesized that circulating IBU levels may be sufficient to decrease bilirubin glucuronidation compensating the decrease in TBC. Indeed, competitive inhibition of bilirubin glucuronidation by 15–30% between IBU and bilirubin has been shown in human liver microsomes [41]. In these retrospective studies on two cohorts in 2 separate periods, the increase in TBC could be attributed to several other confounding factors given the duration of the observation period, and the absence of a chronological relationship between study drug administration and peak TBC. Van Overmeire et al. reported no change in UB concentrations before and after IBU infusion at the recommended dose regimen in 15 preterm neonates [42]. However, Aranda et al. showed significantly higher UB in 113

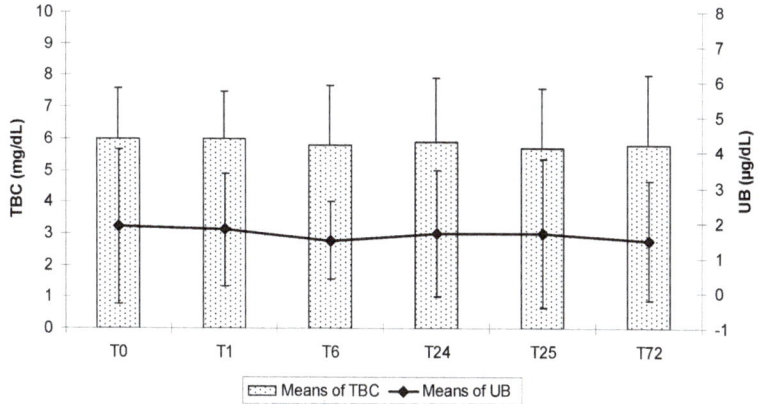

🔲 Fig. 5.3. Mean TBC and UB concentrations during IBU course. T-bar represent 1 SD. Blood samples were taken before (T0), 1 h after (T1) and 6 h after the loading dose of IBU (T6), before (T24) and 1 h after (T25) the first maintenance dose and 72 h after (T72) the beginning of treatment.

IBU-treated newborns without a correlation between IBU concentrations and UB [43].

The preliminary results of a monocenter prospective study specifically designed to evaluate whether the current dosing schedule of IBU (10–5–5 mg/kg every 24 h) may interfere with bilirubin-albumin binding have been reported at the PAS annual meeting [37]. Thirty-four premature newborns with a gestational age below 32 weeks were included. Individual serial blood samples were taken before (T0), 1 h (T1) and 6 h (T6) after the loading dose, before (T24) and 1 h (T25) after the second dose and 72 h (T72) after starting IBU. TBC and UB levels were assayed by the modified peroxidase method and IBU concentration were measured using chiral high-pressure liquid chromatography. At inclusion, all patients had a TBC below 10 mg/dL and were relatively stable during the course of IBU treatment. No significant changes in UB were observed after the administration of IBU (🔲 Fig. 5.3). IBU dosages showed close mean plasmatic peaks after the first and 2nd injection of IBU (56.6 ± 22.1 μg/mL and 49.1 ± 12.9 μg/mL, respectively). However, there was a large interindividual variability of IBU levels after the loading dose (from 18.9 μg/l to 122.7 μg/l). There was no correlation between the increase in

IBU levels and the changes of UB. Moreover, no altered auditory brainstem response could be detected at 36 weeks and no clinical signs of bilirubin neurotoxicity could be detected in the surviving infants. No significant bilirubin displacement could be observed after intravenous administration of IBU at the current dosing schedule (10–5–5 mg/kg/day). However, this study does not provide information about possible risks of IBU use when the bilirubin levels are higher than 10 mg/dL or if higher IBU doses are used.

Conclusions

Despite advances in the care of neonates bilirubin encephalopathy (kernicterus) remains a difficult problem, particularly in preterm infants. For a given TBC, the concentration of UB may increase when the bilirubin binding capacity of albumin is exceeded or when substances compete for its binding sites on albumin. IBU is widely used for the treatment of hsPDA in preterm newborns. It is highly bound to albumin (95%) and displaces bilirubin from albumin binding sites at high IBU concentrations in vitro. The first results in vivo seem to demonstrate that the risk of bilirubin encephalopathy is not increased with IBU at the current dosing scheme of 10–5–5 mg/kg and when the TBC is below 10 mg/dL. Despite these reassuring results, caution should always be paid in order to achieve as low as possible bilirubin levels at the time of IBU administration and if higher IBU doses are used.

References

1. The Vermont-Oxford Trials Network (1993) Very low birth weight outcomes for 1990. Investigators of the Vermont-Oxford Trials Network Database Project. Pediatrics 91: 540–545
2. Mosca F, Bray M, Lattanzio M, Fumagalli M, Tosetto C (1997) Comparative evaluation of the effects of indomethacin and ibuprofen on cerebral perfusion and oxygenation in preterm infants with patent ductus arteriosus. J Pediatr 131: 549–554
3. Pezzati M, Vangi V, Biagiotti R, Bertini G, Cianciulli D, Rubaltelli FF (1999) Effects of indomethacin and ibuprofen on mesenteric and renal blood flow in preterm infants with patent ductus arteriosus. J Pediatr 135: 733–738
4. Cooper-Peel C, Brodersen R, Robertson A (1996) Does ibuprofen affect bilirubin-albumin binding in newborn infant serum? Pharmacol Toxicol 79: 297–299
5. Ahlfors CE (2004) Effect of ibuprofen on bilirubin-albumin binding. J Pediatr 144: 386–388

6. Ambat MT, Ostrea EM Jr, Aranda JV (2008) Effect of ibuprofen L-lysinate on bilirubin binding to albumin as measured by saturation index and horseradish peroxidase assays. J Perinatol 28: 287–290

7. Soligard HT, Nilsen OG, Bratlid D (2010) Displacement of bilirubin from albumin by Ibuprofen in vitro. Pediatr Res 67: 614–618

8. Brodersen R, Ebbesen F (1983) Bilirubin-displacing effect of ampicillin, indomethacin, chlorpromazine, gentamicin, and parabens in vitro and in newborn infants. J Pharm Sci 72: 248–253

9. Bhutani VK, Johnson LH, Shapiro SM (2004) Kernicterus in sick and preterm infants (1999–2002): a need for an effective preventive approach. Semin Perinatol 28: 319–325

10. Okumura A, Kidokoro H, Shoji H, Nakazawa T, Mimaki M, Fujii K, Oba H, Shimizu T (2009) Kernicterus in preterm infants. Pediatrics 123: e1052–1058

11. Oh W, Tyson JE, Fanaroff AA et al. (2003) Association between peak serum bilirubin and neurodevelopmental outcomes in extremely low birth weight infants. Pediatrics 112: 773–779

12. van de Bor M, Ens-Dokkum M, Schreuder AM, Veen S, Brand R, Verloove-Vanhorick SP (1992) Hyperbilirubinemia in low birth weight infants and outcome at 5 years of age. Pediatrics 89: 359–364

13. Wennberg RP, Ahlfors CE, Bhutani VK, Johnson LH, Shapiro SM (2006) Toward understanding kernicterus: a challenge to improve the management of jaundiced newborns. Pediatrics 117: 474–485

14. Cashore WJ, Oh W (1982) Unbound bilirubin and kernicterus in low-birth-weight infants. Pediatrics 69: 481–485

15. Ahlfors CE, Amin SB, Parker AE (2009) Unbound bilirubin predicts abnormal automated auditory brainstem response in a diverse newborn population. J Perinatol 29: 305–309

16. Cashore WJ (1980) Free bilirubin concentrations and bilirubin-binding affinity in term and preterm infants. J Pediatr 96: 521–527

17. Bender GJ, Cashore WJ, Oh W (2007) Ontogeny of bilirubin-binding capacity and the effect of clinical status in premature infants born at less than 1300 grams. Pediatrics 120: 1067–1073

18. Ebbesen F, Nyboe J (1983) Postnatal changes in the ability of plasma albumin to bind bilirubin. Acta Paediatr Scand 72: 665–670

19. Watchko JF (2006) Kernicterus and the molecular mechanisms of bilirubin-induced CNS injury in newborns. Neuromolecular Med 8: 513–529

20. Hansen TW (2000) Bilirubin oxidation in brain. Mol Genet Metab 71: 411–417

21. Hanko E, Tommarello S, Watchko JF, Hansen TW (2003) Administration of drugs known to inhibit P-glycoprotein increases brain bilirubin and alters the regional distribution of bilirubin in rat brain. Pediatr Res 54: 441–445

22. Jacobsen J, Wennberg RP (1974) Determination of unbound bilirubin in the serum of newborns. Clin Chem 20: 783

23. Ahlfors CE, Vreman HJ, Wong RJ, Bender GJ, Oh W, Morris BH, Stevenson DK (2007) Effects of sample dilution, peroxidase concentration, and chloride ion on the measurement of unbound bilirubin in premature newborns. Clin Biochem 40: 261–267

24. Ahlfors CE (2000) Measurement of plasma unbound unconjugated bilirubin. Anal Biochem 279: 130–135
25. Ahlfors CE (2000) Unbound bilirubin associated with kernicterus: a historical approach. J Pediatr 137: 540–544
26. Robertson A, Karp W, Brodersen R (1991) Bilirubin displacing effect of drugs used in neonatology. Acta Paediatr Scand 80: 1119–1127
27. Silverman WA, Andersen DH, Blanc WA, Crozier DN (1956) A difference in mortality rate and incidence of kernicterus among premature infants alloted to two prophylactic antibacterial regimens. Pediatrics 18: 614–625
28. Shimabuku R, Nakamura H, Matsuo T (1983) Effect of Sulfisoxazole on Bilirubin-Albumin Binding in Gunn Rats. Acta Paediatr Jpn 25: 304–308
29. Starinsky R, Shafrir E (1970) Displacement of albumin-bound bilirubin by free fatty acids. Implications for neonatal hyperbilirubinemia. Clin Chim Acta 29: 311–318
30. Aranda JV, Varvarigou A, Beharry K, Bansal R, Bardin C, Modanlou H, Papageorgiou A, Chemtob S (1997) Pharmacokinetics and protein binding of intravenous ibuprofen in the premature newborn infant. Acta Paediatr 86: 289–293
31. Aranda JV, Clyman R, Cox B et al. (2009) A randomized, double-blind, placebo-controlled trial on intravenous ibuprofen L-lysine for the early closure of nonsymptomatic patent ductus arteriosus within 72 hours of birth in extremely low-birth-weight infants. Am J Perinatol 26: 235–245
32. Desfrere L, Zohar S, Morville P, Brunhes A, Chevret S, Pons G, Moriette G, Rey E, Treluyer JM (2005) Dose-finding study of ibuprofen in patent ductus arteriosus using the continual reassessment method. J Clin Pharm Ther 30: 121–132
33. Gregoire N, Desfrere L, Roze JC, Kibleur Y, Koehne P (2008) Population pharmacokinetic analysis of ibuprofen enantiomers in preterm newborn infants. J Clin Pharmacol 48: 1460–1468
34. Van Overmeire B, Touw D, Schepens PJ, Kearns GL, van den Anker JN (2001) Ibuprofen pharmacokinetics in preterm infants with patent ductus arteriosus. Clin Pharmacol Ther 70: 336–343
35. Pees C, Walch A, Koehne P (2010) Echocardiography predicts closure of patent ductus arteriosus in response to ibuprofen in infants less than 28 week gestational age. Early Hum Dev 86: 503–508
36. Gournay V, Roze JC, Kuster A et al. (2004) Prophylactic ibuprofen versus placebo in very premature infants: a randomised, double-blind, placebo-controlled trial. Lancet 364: 1939–1944
37. Desfrere L, Mourdie J, Barbier A, Moriette G (2007) Effect of Ibuprofen on Unbound Bilirubin Levels in Preterm Newborns. PAS Annual Meeting, Toronto, Canada
38. Diot C, Kibleur Y, Desfrere L (2010) Effect of ibuprofen on bilirubin-albumin binding in vitro at concentrations observed during treatment of patent ductus arteriosus. Early Hum Dev 86: 315–317
39. Koehne PS, Huseman D, Walch E, Schuelke M, Varon R, Karbasiyan M, Aust G, Obladen M (2006) Genetic deafness in a preterm infant with a critical postnatal course. Pediatr Crit Care Med 7: 270–272

40. Rheinlaender C, Helfenstein D, Walch E, Berns M, Obladen M, Koehne P (2009) Total serum bilirubin levels during cyclooxygenase inhibitor treatment for patent ductus arteriosus in preterm infants. Acta Paediatr 98: 36–42

41. Kuehl A, Lampe JW, Potter JD, Bigler J (2005) Glucuronidation of non-steroidal anti-inflammatory drugs: identifying the enzymes responsible in human liver microsomes. Drug Metab Dispos 33: 1027–1035

42. Van Overmeire B, Vanhagendoren S, Schepens P, Ahlfors C (2004) The influence of Ibuprofen-lysine on unbound bilirubin plasma levels in preterm neonates [Abstract]. PAS Annual Meeting, San Francisco, CA

43. Aranda JV, Wrong RJ, Thomas R, Vreman HJ, Steinhilber G, Ahlfors C, Stevenson DK (2008) Plasma unbound bilirubin in placebo and ibuprofen treated preterm neonates [Abstract]. PAS Annual Meeting, Honolulu, Hawaii

Controversies Around Treatment of the Open Duct

B. Van Overmeire

Introduction

The optimal management of a patent ductus arteriosus (PDA) in the preterm infant is an ongoing debate which is fueled by changing clinical evidence, new insights in pathophysiology, and also influenced by the appearance of additional therapies in ante- and postnatal care during the last decade. Wide variability exists in the treatment approach of the PDA: e.g. the postnatal age at which the first dose of drug is given (prophylaxis, early or late treatment), the amount of fluids administered, which drug to use, additional courses or other adapted dosing schemes, and finally in last years the question arises more and more frequently whether any treatment at all is necessary in very low birth weight infants (VLBW). This chapter aims to address some of the current controversies.

Fluid Restriction for PDA?

It is common belief that excessive fluid administration during the first days of life in VLBW infants is associated with an increased risk of developing a PDA [1]. Unfortunately, poor solid evidence exists to support this view. Clear guidelines for fluid therapy in this group of patients are not well defined. Many authors have recommended to restrict the fluid intake to allow a negative water balance in the first week of life. A systematic meta-analysis on this topic was last updated in 2008 and is based on 5 studies that presented data in 7 to 9 publications [2]. Four of 5 included trials are dating from the era before antenatal steroids and exogenous surfactant therapy [1, 3–5]. Moreover, only a study of Bell from 1980 showed convincing evidence that restricted water intake was associated with less PDA. The meta-analysis including the four trials in which data were presented with regard to PDA (Bell 1980 [1], Lorenz 1982 [3], Tammela 1992 [4] and Kavvadia 1999 [6]) showed an overall reduced risk of PDA when water restriction was applied (risk ratio: 0.52 (95% confidence interval [CI]: 0.37–0.73)). Based on this analysis the number needed to treat with restricted water intake to prevent one case of PDA is 7 (95% CI: 5–14). The authors conclude that the practice of restricting water intake to physiological needs without allowing dehydration in preterm infants might be expected to decrease the risk of PDA [2].

Additional information comes from the study of Stephens in 2008 [7]. In a group of 204 extremely low birth weight infants, an increased risk of PDA and BPD was associated with high fluid intake as assessed by logistic regression analysis while controlling for confounding variables. They calculated that a fluid intake above 170 mL/kg/day on day 3 alone was associated with an increased risk of PDA, suggesting that restriction to less than this value is not warranted. On the other hand, limiting water intake when a baby has a hemodynamically significant PDA may lead to reduced stroke volume, cardiac output and may further compromise tissue perfusion [8].

Which Drug Should Be Used?

Until 2004, indomethacin was the only COX inhibitor approved for treatment of PDA in most countries. Other non-steroidal anti-inflammatory drugs (NSAIDs) have been used with varying successes. The fewer side effects of aspirin were irrelevant as these seemed to be associated with lower efficacy [9]. Ethamsylate has been used in preventive approach but never gained widespread use [10]. Since the late 1990s ibuprofen has been studied as an alternative for the treatment and prophylaxis of PDA and it has now been extensively compared to indomethacin [11, 12]. Ibuprofen disturbs significantly less regional circulations, which may offer less dysfunction of kidney, intestines, and brain [13, 14]. Urine production was less affected in preterm infants (n=148) that were treated with ibuprofen on day 2 or 3 of life as compared to those receiving indomethacin [15], an observation which made ibuprofen to be introduced for clinical use in preterm infants. Necrotizing enterocolitis was diagnosed twice as often in the indomethacin group (8 vs. 4; p=0.37) [15]. Cerebral oxygen availability has repeatedly been shown to be less affected with ibuprofen [14, 16]. Systematic reviews of the trials that evaluated indomethacin or ibuprofen for early treatment of a non-symptomatic or symptomatic PDA confirmed a comparable efficacy of both drugs [17]. The most recently updated systematic meta-analysis included twenty studies [18]. There was no statistically significant difference between indomethacin and ibuprofen efficacy or in failure to close the ductus in 19 comparative studies including 956 infants with a typical relative risk (RR) of 0.94 (95% CI: 0.76–1.17). Infants receiving ibuprofen treatment have less evidence of transient renal failure and less risk of developing necrotizing enterocolitis: 15 studies including 865 infants; typical RR 0.68 (95% CI: 0.47–0.99). No other differences were noted, e.g. mortality, reopening of the ductus, need for ligation, duration of ventilatory support, duration of supplementary oxygen nor development of BPD. Indomethacin and ibuprofen are administered following different dosing schemes as a result of their distinct pharmacokinetic profiles. Prolonged dosing schedules have been tried to augment efficacy/side effect ratio of indomethacin, and more recently of ibuprofen. Up to now this has not been convincingly efficient [19].

A Choice Based on Side Effects?

Due to their vasoconstrictive effects, both indomethacin and ibuprofen affect the perfusion of various organ systems e.g. the gut, kidney and brain. Although ibuprofen initially seemed to have a more favourable safety profile with less disturbance of regional circulations [11–16], the occurrence of unexpected hypoxemia caused a lot of concern. Acute pulmonary hypertension developed in 3 preterm infants immediately after the infusion of ibuprofen THAM-buffered solution [20]. A clear explanation for this phenomenon is lacking. In another study, 169 infants were treated with ibuprofen-lysine and one presented the same adverse effect [21]. No causal relationship could be found between 2 cases of PPHN and ibuprofen-lysine in another 229 treated infants, PPHN occurred in both the ibuprofen and control groups [22]. Additional trials did not confirm an association between the use of ibuprofen-lysine and severe hypoxemia. Although the trial that first reported PPHN as serious adverse effect was halted by the French authorities [23], the ibuprofen formulation under investigation became registered for clinical use in Europe in 2004. Ibuprofen-lysine was registered for treatment and prophylaxis of PDA in preterm infants in the US in 2006.

Ibuprofen is insoluble in water and more than 90% bound to serum albumin [24]. An in-vitro model demonstrated that at higher ibuprofen concentrations (750 μmol/L or 150 mg/L) in infant serum containing bilirubin, the fraction of unbound bilirubin increases fourfold [25]. This displacement of bilirubin from albumin binding sites may be clinically relevant in jaundiced preterm infants, as high levels of free bilirubin are associated with brain damage, hearing loss and kernicterus [26, 27]. When ibuprofen is administered in the recommended dosage of 10, 5 and 5 mg/kg at 24 hourly intervals to neonatal infants, ibuprofen serum peak levels of 20 to 40 mg/L are reached [28]. According to the in-vitro model, an increase of 10% of the free fraction of bilirubin can be expected at such ibuprofen levels. Three smaller studies exploring the rise of unbound bilirubin were rather reassuring in this respect [29–31].

The occurrence of an isolated ileal perforation is an additional risk of the use of NSAIDs for closing PDA in preterm infants, particularly when there is concomitant use of steroids [32, 33]. Although predominantly reported for indomethacin, this risk may be similar for ibuprofen as its mechanism is related to microvascular changes and not to disturbances of the regional perfusion of the gut [34]. Increased bleeding tendency has been described after indomethacin use [35], but except from some increased occult blood appearing in stools this does not seem to cause clinically relevant problems. Some neonatal intensive care units are reluctant to continue or introduce enteral feedings during NSAIDs treatment. Almost eighty percent of the infants that participated in the European trials of prophylactic and early therapeutic NSAIDs for PDA were receiving trophic feedings without any apparent untoward effect [15, 23, 36, 37]. The most recent meta-analysis showed that necrotizing enterocolitis is less likely to occur post ibuprofen than post indomethacin treatment [18].

Optimal Dosing of Indomethacin and Ibuprofen?

Pharmacokinetic parameters vary widely in preterm infants due to physiological changes that occur after birth. Studies have shown largely prolonged half-life for indomethacin (11–36 h) and reduced clearance rate in the preterm infant. Both parameters reveal marked interindividual variations [38, 39]. The volume of distribution also varies and is itself influenced by the patency of the ductus [40]. Accordingly, optimal therapeutic dosing is difficult to establish [41]. The most commonly used doses for indomethacin are 3 times 0.1 to 0.25 mg/kg administered every 12 to 24 hours. The lower dose with longer interval is recommended when treatment is initiated on the first day. The registered dosing scheme for ibuprofen consists of a first dose of 10 mg/kg followed by a second and third dose of 5 mg/kg at 24 hourly intervals.

In order to improve efficacy/side effect ratio of NSAIDs during treatment for PDA, a variety of adapted dosing schemes have been studied. As it has been observed that PGE_2 production resurges within 5 days of indomethacin treatment [42], a prolonged course consisting of additional indomethacin doses has been tried [19]. Unfortunately, no significant benefit for closure rates, not less reopenings or ligations, and no improvement for BPD, IVH or mortality rates has been obtained. A lower proportion of infants with diminished urine output was observed (typical RR 0.27; 95%CI: 0.13–0.6) but at the expense of an increased risk of NEC (RR 1.87; 95% CI: 1.07–3.27) [19].

The continuous infusion of indomethacin has been advocated to avoid disturbances in cerebral perfusion [43], but was reported later to be less effective in extremely low birth weight infants [44]. Interestingly, by applying a stepwise increasing indomethacin dosage based on echocardiographic evaluation, the group of Sperandio et al. obtained ductal closure rates up to 98% without apparently increasing side effects. After an initial standard treatment, subsequent doses were given if the ductus persisted as assessed by Doppler echocardiography. Cumulative indomethacin doses were as high as 6 mg/kg [45]. Unfortunately, their findings were based on a retrospective chart review and have not yet been confirmed in a blinded prospective setting. On the contrary, Jegatheesan and collaborators reported only little effect on closure rates by increasing indomethacin doses up to 0.5 mg/kg in their multicenter randomized controlled trial, but observed more renal side effects and a higher incidence of moderate and severe retinopathy of prematurity [46]. As the efficacy of ibuprofen at extremely low gestational ages is comparably reduced to indomethacin [47], the administration of additional doses has been investigated. In a group of 25 VLBW infants that received a second course of 3 doses of ibuprofen the additional closure was 48% [48]. Su et al. obtained an additional closure rate of 50% by administrating up to 6 doses of ibuprofen [47]. Similar efficacy was demonstrated after the first and second course in a study population of 160 infants with a birth weight below 1000 g with a cumulative closure rate of 65% [49]. In order to optimize the efficacy of ibuprofen, an adapted dosing scheme based on postnatal age has been proposed. In order to achieve optimal concentrations (AUC: area under the curve) irrespective of the gestational age at birth, three administrations at 24 h intervals were recommended with the conventional dose of 10–5–5 mg/kg for patients up to 70 h after birth, 14–7–7 mg/kg for infants between 70 and 108 h of life, and 18–9–9 mg/kg for patients between 108 and 180 h of life [50]. Further studies are warranted to investigate whether an individualized ibuprofen dosing scheme would result in an increased benefit/risk ratio.

Is There a Role for Prophylaxis?

A vast amount of studies has investigated the timing of pharmacological treatment of PDA. Prophylactic, early pre-symptomatic and symptomatic treatment strategies have been compared [51]. More than 30 studies and reviews addressed prophylaxis with NSAIDs in preterm infants. The last updated meta-analyses available demonstrate that both prophylactic indomethacin and ibuprofen reduce significantly the risk of developing a symptomatic PDA and the need for ductal ligation [52, 53]. Nineteen prophylactic indomethacin trials were eligible in which 2872 infants were included. The incidence of symptomatic PDA was very significantly reduced: typical RR 0.44; 95% CI: 0.38–0.50. In the studies eligible for the ibuprofen review the ductus had closed spontaneously in 60% of the infants of the control group by the third day of life. Based on available data the prophylactic administration of ibuprofen cannot be recommended. Indomethacin offers the additional effect of reducing the occurrence of intraventricular hemorrhage (typical RR 0.66; 95% CI: 0.53–0.82). No positive effect on any other outcome parameter could be demonstrated. In particular no decrease in the rates of bronchopulmonary dysplasia, death, necrotizing enterocolitis, or white matter disease. Notwithstanding the decrease of IVH, an improved neurodevelopmental outcome has not been demonstrated [53, 54].

Conclusion

Although several controversies remain about management of a PDA, moderate changes in approach are described. Limiting fluid administration below 170 ml/kg/day seems definitely associated with less PDA. Based on cumulative evidence, the efficacy of indomethacin and ibuprofen in closing the ductus is comparable. The last one seems to have a more favourable safety profile for now. Adapted dosing schemes may increase closure rates, but studies confirming a safe higher dosing of ibuprofen should be awaited.

References

1. Bell EF, Warburton D, Stonestreet BS, Oh W (1980) Effect of fluid administration on the development of symptomatic patent ductus arteriosus and congestive heart failure in premature infants. N Engl J Med 302: 598–604
2. Bell EF, Acarregui MJ (2008) Restricted versus liberal water intake for preventing morbidity and mortality in preterm infants. Cochrane Database Syst Rev 1: CD000503
3. Lorenz JM, Kleinman LI, Kotagal UR, Reller MD (1982) Water balance in very low-birth-weight infants: relationship to water and sodium intake and effect on outcome. J Pediatr 101: 423–432
4. Tammela OK, Lanning FP, Koivisto ME (1992) The relationship of fluid restriction during the 1st month of life to the occurrence and severity of bronchopulmonary dysplasia in low birth weight infants: a 1-year radiological follow up. Eur J Pediatr 51: 295–299
5. von Stockhausen HB, Struve M (1980) Effects of highly varying parenteral fluid intakes in premature and newborn infants during the first three days of life. Klin Padiatr 192: 539–546
6. Kavvadia V, Greenough A, Dimitriou G, Hooper R, Kavvadia V, Greenough A, Dimitriou G, Hooper R (2000) Randomised trial of fluid restriction in ventilated very low birthweight infants. Arch Dis Child Fetal Neonatal Ed 83: F91–96
7. Stephens BE, Gargus RA, Walden RV, Mance M, Nye J, McKinley L, Tucker R, Vohr BR (2008) Fluid regimens in the first week of life may increase risk of patent ductus arteriosus in extremely low birth weight infants. J Perinatol 28: 123–128
8. Teixeira LS, Shivananda SP, Stephens D, Van Arsdell G, McNamara PJ (2008) Postoperative cardiorespiratory instability following ligation of the preterm ductus arteriosus is related to early need for intervention. J Perinatol 28: 803–810
9. Van Overmeire B, Brus F, van Acker K J, van der Auwera J C, Schasfoort M, Elzenga N J, Okken A (1995) Aspirin versus indomethacin treatment of patent ductus arteriosus in preterm infants with respiratory distress syndrome. Pediatr Res 38: 886–891
10. Amato M, Hüppi P, Markus D (1993) Prevention of symptomatic patent ductus arteriosus with ethamsylate in babies treated with exogenous surfactant. J Perinatol 13: 2–7
11. Van Overmeire B, Follens I, Hartmann S, Creten WL, Van Acker KJ (1997) Treatment of patent ductus arteriosus with ibuprofen. Arch Dis Child 76: F179–F184
12. Varvarigou A, Bardin CL, Beharry K, Chemtob S, Papageorgiou A, Aranda JV (1996) Early ibuprofen administration to prevent patent ductus arteriosus in premature newborn infants. JAMA 275: 539–544
13. Pezzati M, Vangi V, Biagiotti R et al. (1999) Effects of indomethacin and ibuprofen on mesenteric and renal blood flow in preterm infants with patent ductus arteriosus. J Pediatr 135: 733–738
14. Patel J, Roberts I, Azzopardi D et al. (2000) Randomized double-blind controlled trial comparing the effects of ibuprofen with indomethacin on cerebral hemodynamics in preterm infants with patent ductus arteriosus. Pediatr Res 47: 36–42
15. Van Overmeire B, Smets K, Lecoutere D, Van de Broek H, Weyler J, De Groote K, Langhendries J-P (2000) A comparison of ibuprofen and indomethacin for closure of patent ductus arteriosus. N Engl J Med 343: 674–681

16. Mosca F, Bray M, Lattanzio M et al. (1997) Comparative evaluation of the effects of indomethacin and ibuprofen on cerebral perfusion and oxygenation in preterm infants with patent ductus arteriosus. J Pediatr 131: 549–554

17. Thomas RL, Parker GC, Van Overmeire B, Aranda JV (2005) A meta-analysis of ibuprofen versus indomethacin for closure of patent ductus arteriosus. Eur J Pediatr 164: 135–140

18. Ohlsson A, Walia R, Shah S (2010) Ibuprofen for the treatment of patent ductus arteriosus in preterm and/or low birth weight infants. Cochrane Database Syst Rev 4: CD003481

19. Herrera C, Holberton J, Davis P (2007) Prolonged versus short course of indomethacin for the treatment of patent ductus arteriosus in preterm infants. Cochrane Database Syst Rev 2: CD003480

20. Gournay V, Savagner C, Thiriez G, Kuster A, Rozé J-C (2002) Pulmonary hypertension after ibuprofen prophylaxis in very preterm infants. Lancet 359: 1486–1488

21. Mosca F, Bray M, Stucchi I, Fumagalli M (2002) Pulmonary hypertension after ibuprofen prophylaxis in very preterm infants. Lancet 360: 1023–1024

22. Aranda JV, Clyman R, Cox B et al. (2009) A randomized, double-blind, placebo-controlled trial on intravenous ibuprofen L-lysine for the early closure of nonsymptomatic patent ductus arteriosus within 72 hours of birth in extremely low-birth-weight infants. Am J Perinatol 26: 235–245

23. Gournay V, Roze JC, Kuster A et al. (2004) Prophylactic ibuprofen versus placebo in very premature infants: a randomised, double-blind, placebo-controlled trial. Lancet 364: 1939–1944

24. Aranda JV, Varvarigou A, Beharry K, Bansal R, Bardin C, Modanlou H, Papageorgiou A, Chemtob S (1997) Pharmacokinetics and protein binding of intravenous ibuprofen in the premature newborn infant. Acta Paediatr 86: 289–293

25. Cooper-Peel C, Brodersen R, Robertson A (1996) Does ibuprofen affect bilirubin-albumin binding in newborn infant serum? Pharmacol Toxicol 79: 297–299

26. Ahlfors CE (2004) Effect of ibuprofen on bilirubin-albumin binding. J Pediatr 144: 386–388

27. Ahlfors CE, Marshall GD, Wolcott DK, Olson DC, Van Overmeire B (2006) Measurement of unbound bilirubin by the peroxidase test using zone fluidics. Clinica Chimica Acta 365: 78–85

28. Van Overmeire B, Touw D, Schepens PJC, Kearns GL, van den Anker JN (2001) Ibuprofen pharmacokinetics in preterm infants with patent ductus arteriosus. Clin Pharmacol Ther 70: 336–343

29. Van Overmeire B, Vanhagendoren S, Schepens PJ, Ahlfors CE (2004) The influence of ibuprofen-lysine on unbound bilirubin plasma levels in preterm neonates. Pediatr Res 55: 474A

30. Desfrere L, Zohar S, Morville P, Brunhes A, Chevret S, Pons G, Moriette G, Rey E, Treluyer JM (2005) Dose-finding study of ibuprofen in patent ductus arteriosus using the continual reassessment method. J Clin Pharm Ther 30: 121–132

31. Diot C, Kibleur Y, Desfrere L (2010) Effect of ibuprofen on bilirubin-albumin binding in vitro at concentrations observed during treatment of patent ductus arteriosus. Early Hum Dev 86: 315–317

6

32. Watterberg KL, Gerdes JS, Cole CH et al. (2004) Prophylaxis of early adrenal insufficiency to prevent bronchopulmonary dysplasia: a multicenter trial. Pediatrics 114: 1649–1657

33. Paquette L, Friedlich P, Ramanathan R, Seri I (2006) Concurrent use of indomethacin and dexamethasone increases the risk of spontaneous intestinal perforation in very low birth weight neonates. J Perinatol 26: 486–492

34. Tatli MM, Kumral A, Duman N, Demir K, Gurcu O, Ozkan H (2004) Spontaneous intestinal perforation after oral ibuprofen treatment of patent ductus arteriosus in two very-low-birthweight infants. Acta Paediatr 93: 999–1001

35. Corazza MS, Davis RF, Merrit TA, Bejar R, Cvetnic W (1984) Prolonged bleeding time in preterm infants receiving indomethacin for patent ductus arteriosus. J Pediatr 105: 292–296

36. Van Overmeire B, Van de Broek H, Van Laer P, Weyler J, Vanhaesebrouck P (2001) Early versus late indomethacin treatment for patent ductus arteriosus in premature infants with respiratory distress syndrome. J Pediatr 138: 205–211

37. Van Overmeire B, Allegaert K, Casaer A, Debauche C, Decaluwé W, Jespers A, Weyler J, Harrewijn I, Langhendries JP and the MIPS investigators (2004) Prophylactic ibuprofen in premature infants: a multicentre, randomised, double-blind, placebo-controlled trial. Lancet 364: 1945–1944

38. Thalji AA, Carr I, Yeh TF, Raval D, Luken JA, Pildes RS (1980) Pharmacokinetics of intravenously administered indomethacin in premature infants. J Pediatr 97: 995–1000

39. Shaffer CL, Gal P, Ransom JL, Carlos RQ, Smith MS, Davey AM, Dimaguila MA, Brown YL, Schall SA (2002) Effect of age and birth weight on indomethacin pharmacodynamics in neonates treated for patent ductus arteriosus. Crit Care Med 30: 343–348

40. Gal P, Ransom JL, Weaver RL, Schall S, Wyble LE, Carlos RQ, Brown Y (1991) Indomethacin pharmacokinetics in neonates: the value of volume of distribution as a marker of permanent patent ductus arteriosus closure. Ther Drug Monit 13: 42–45

41. Guimarães H, Rocha G, Tomé T, Anatolitou F, Sarafidis K, Fanos V (2009) Non-steroid anti-inflammatory drugs in the treatment of patent ductus arteriosus in European newborns. J Matern Fetal Neonatal Med 22 (Suppl 3): 77–80

42. Seyberth HW (1983) Effect of prolonged indomethacin therapy on renal function and selected vasoactive hormones in VLBW infants with symptomatic patent ductus arteriosus. J Pediatr 103: 979–984

43. Christmann V, Liem KD, Semmekrot BA, van de Bor M (2002) Changes in cerebral, renal and mesenteric blood flow velocity during continuous and bolus infusion of indomethacin. Acta Paediatr 91: 440–446

44. de Vries NK, Jagroep FK, Jaarsma AS, Elzenga NJ, Bos AF (2005) Continuous indomethacin infusion may be less effective than bolus infusions for ductal closure in very low birth weight infants. Am J Perinatol 22: 71–75

45. Sperandio M, Beedgen B, Feneberg R, Huppertz C, Brüssau J, Pöschl J, Linderkamp O (2005) Effectiveness and side effects of an escalating, stepwise approach to indomethacin treatment for symptomatic patent ductus arteriosus in premature infants below 33 weeks of gestation. Pediatrics 116: 1361–1366

46. Jegatheesan P, Ianus V, Buchh B (2008) Increased indomethacin dosing for persistent patent ductus arteriosus in preterm infants: a multicenter, randomized, controlled trial. J Pediatr 153: 183–189

47. Su BH, Lin HC, Chiun HY, Hsieh HY, Chen HH, Tsai YC (2008) Comparison of ibuprofen and indomethacin for early-targeted treatment of patent ductus arteriosus in extremely premature infants: A randomized controlled trial. Arch Dis Child 93: F94–99

48. Lago P, Bettiol T, Salvadori S, Pitassi I, Vianello A, Chiandetti L, Saia OS (2002) Safety and efficacy of ibuprofen versus indomethacin in preterm infants treated for patent ductus arteriosus: a randomised controlled trial. Eur J Pediatr 161: 202–207

49. Richards J, Johnson A, Fox G, Campbell M (2009) A second course of ibuprofen is effective in the closure of a clinically significant PDA in ELBW infants. Pediatrics 124: e287–292

50. Hirt D, Van Overmeire B, Treluyer JM, Langhendries JP, Marguglio A, Eisinger MJ, Schepens P, Urien S (2008) An optimized ibuprofen dosing scheme for preterm neonates with patent ductus arteriosus, based on a population pharmacokinetic and pharmacodynamic study. Br J Clin Pharmacol 65: 629–636

51. Clyman RI (1996) Recommendations for the postnatal use of indomethacin: An analysis of four separate treatment strategies. J Pediatr 128: 601–607

52. Shah S, Ohlsson A (2006) Ibuprofen for the prevention of patent ductus arteriosus in preterm and/or low birth weight infants. Cochrane Database Syst Rev 1: CD004213

53. Fowlie PW, Davis PG, McGuire W (2010) Prophylactic intravenous indomethacin for preventing mortality and morbidity in preterm infants. Cochrane Database Syst Rev 7: CD000174

54. Schmidt B, Davis P, Moddemann D, Ohlsson A, Roberts RS, Saigal S, Solimano A,Vincer M, Wright LL, for the Trial of Indomethacin Prophylaxis in Preterms Investigators (2001) Long-term effects of indomethacin prophylaxis in extremely-low-birth-weight infants. N Engl J Med 344: 1966–1972

High-Dose Therapy with Cyclooxygenase-Inhibitors for Symptomatic Persistent Ductus Arteriosus in Preterms

B. Beedgen

Persistens of the ductus arteriosus in preterms is a common problem. Especially patients with respiratory distress syndrome are affected. A ductus that is patent >72 h can be considered as persistent. Approximately 30% of infants below 1500 g and 50–70% below 1000 g are affected [1, 2]. A significant left-to-right shunt over the ductus leads to systemic hypoperfusion and pulmonary hyperperfusion. Possible consequences are increased mortality, cardiac failure, renal failure, necrotizing entercolitis (NEC), intraventricular hemorrhage (IVH), pulmonary edema with prolonged ventilation, increased oxygen requirement, and bronchopulmonary dysplasia (BPD).

Treatment Options

Once the diagnosis is confirmed, controversies exist about the treatment of choice. Treatment options include conservative medical management, prophylactic or therapeutic pharmacological therapy with cyclooxygenase inhibitors (indomethacin or ibuprofen) or surgical ligation. Recent surveys of PDA management in the USA and Australia indicated a wide practice variation [3, 4].

Conservative management is an option if PDA is not symptomatic. This approach is associated with a high failure rate, especially in very low birth weight infants. An asymptomatic PDA still patent at discharge closes in 85% of cases without further treatment [5]. Surgical ligation involves thoracotomy and is associated with such acute morbidities as pneumothorax, chylothorax, laryngeal nerve palsy, respiratory compromise and blood pressure fluctuations. Recent publications show an increased rate of BPD, retinopathy of prematurity (ROP) and severe neurosensory impairment at long-term follow-up after surgical ligation [6, 7]. Therefore, ligation should be considered as last option in selected infants who have failed pharmacological treatment.

Pharmacological Treatment

At the moment, pharmacotherapy seems to be the therapy of choice for safe and effective treatment of significant patent ductus arteriosus (sPDA). Pharmacotherapy uses the cyclooxygenase (COX)-inhibitors indomethacin and ibuprofen. They block the conversion of arachidonic acid to various prostaglandins that are involved in maintaining the patency of the ductus arteriosus. These drugs are chemically different and inhibit COX 1 and 2 isoforms to different degrees. Indomethacin is a stronger COX-1 inhibitor, leading to a decrease in cerebral, gastrointestinal and renal blood flow. This has been attributed to undesirable side effects such as NEC, gastrointestinal perforation and renal failure [14, 15]. Ibuprofen lacks these side effects but has a very high albumin binding affinity, competing with bilirubin binding and so potentially increasing the risk of bilirubin encephalopathy [8]. Cases of pulmonary hypertension and pulmonary hemorrhage have been reported [9].

Optimal timing of pharmacotherapy is still under debate. Treatment options are prophylactic (<24 h), early presymptomatic (days 2–3), therapeutic (days 3–7) or late therapeutic (>7 days) strategy [10].

Prophylactic therapy has shown to reduce the rate of significant PDA and surgical ligation. No changes were seen in the rate of survival, BPD, NEC or ROP. Indomethacin in addition reduces the rate of severe IVH, but disappointingly no long-term benefit regarding neurological and neurodevelopmental outcome was seen [9, 11, 12]. With prophylactic treatment 20–30% of preterms in whom the ductus closes spontaneously in the first 2–3 days are exposed to drugs with possible serious side effects. Because at the moment no evidence-based long-term benefit can be demonstrated, this strategy is not clearly recommended. If prophylactic therapy is done indomethacin is the drug of choice.

Late therapeutic strategy (>7 days) reduces the closure rate [13] and exposes the patient to a long-term hyperperfusion of the lungs and hypoperfusion of vital organs with the potential of increasing the risk for BPD, NEC, IVH and cardiac and renal failure.

At the moment most units use the therapeutic approach with begin of pharmacological therapy between days 3–7. With standard dosing regime of indomethacin (3–6 doses with 0.1–0.2 mg/kg every 12–24 h) and ibuprofen (10–5–5 mg/kg every 24 h) equal closure rates of the ductus arteriosus in about 70% are achieved. Indomethacin seems to result in a higher rate of NEC [15] whereas ibuprofen shows a higher rate of BPD in one meta-analysis [14]. No differences are seen in survival rate or rate of IVH.

Failure rates occur most commonly among infants with either extreme immaturity (<28 weeks of gestation) or advanced postnatal age [13]. Because immature gestation and advanced postnatal age affect both, the volume of distribution and the clearance of indomethacin [16], many investigators have hypothesized that PDA treatment failures may be the result of subtherapeutic plasma indomethacin concentrations [17]. Although no absolute therapeutic range has been defined, as a group, indomethacin treatment failures appear to have lower mean serum concentrations than treatment responders [18]. Jackson et al. proposed that the maintenance of a therapeutic serum level between 475 µg/L to 3500 µg/L over a critical period of 72 hours is essential for the permanent closure of the duct [22]. Non-responders thus may need higher doses of indomethacin. However, there is concern that high doses of indomethacin may increase the risk for severe side effects. Two case reports on indomethacin overdosing in premature infants who were treated for PDA reported only a transient impairment in renal function without any other severe side effects [19, 20]. One of these infants received a 100-fold overdose of indomethacin (20 mg/kg), leading to serum indomethacin levels of almost 10,000 µg/L, which is about 5-fold over the proposed upper limit of the therapeutic range of ~2500 µg/L. The overdose led to the successful closure of the PDA accompanied by transient renal failure, but without other severe side effects. In addition, newborns with hyperprostaglandin-E syndrome where treated in our unit with doses of indomethacin up to 9 mg/kg/day without complications [21].

High-Dose Therapy with Indomethacin

In the early 1990s, we developed a stepwise approach with an escalating indomethacin dosing up to single doses of 1 mg/kg for the 30% of preterms whose PDA did not respond to standard dosing. After diagnosis of sPDA is made between 48 and 72 h of life with echocardiography (ductal diameter ≥1.5 mm, left atrium-to-aortic-root ratio ≥1.3–1.5, decreased diastolic flow in the celiac trunk), infants are treated according to the flowchart shown in ◘ Fig. 7.1. Treatment starts with 0.2 mg/kg indomethacin. Indomethacin (1 mg) is dissolved in normal saline (0.9%) to a final concentration of 0.1 mg/mL and infused over 30 minutes. The same dose is repeated after 12 and 24 hours. Echocardiography is conducted after the third dose. In case of PDA closure or filiform (<1 mm) residual, 2 additional doses at 24 and 48 hours after the third dose complete the standard-dose treatment regimen (◘ Fig. 7.1). In infants where the ductus arteriosus is still significant after the third dose, the single dose of indomethacin is gradually increased by steps of 0.1 mg/kg

Heidelberger algorithm of escalating high-dose therapy with indomethacin for sPDA:

Diagnosis of sPDA (echocardiography in all preterms < 33 weeks between 48 h and 72 h)
indomethacin 0.2 mg/kg iv over 30 min.
reduction of fluid intake to 70% of starting value, aim:stable weight during therapy (to avoid hyponatremia)
same dose after 12 h und 24 h

evaluation of PDA with echocardiography after 36 h

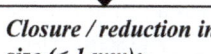

Closure / reduction in size (< 1 mm):

indomethacin 0.2 mg/kg
after 24 h and 48 h

end of therapy

Persistent ductus arteriosus:
daily increase of single dose by 0.1 mg/kg (up to 0,4 mg/kg)
dose in 12 hours intervals (daily echocardiography)

daily increase of single dose by 0.2 mg/kg when single dose ≥ 0.4 mg/kg (maximum single dose 1 mg/kg)
1 mg/kg dose in 12 h - 8 h intervals (daily echocardiography)

Closure / reduction in size (<1 mm):

indomethacin with the same single dose as at closure after 24 h and 48 h (end of therapy)

maximum duration of one course: 7 – 10 days

🔲 Fig. 7.1

per day and given in intervals of 12 hours. Daily echocardiography is performed to monitor the presence of an open ductus. After echocardiographic evidence of a closed ductus, indomethacin is repeated after 24 and 48 hours with the same dose as at closure of the ductus. When the ductus persists after reaching a single dose of 0.4 mg/kg, we continue to increase the single dose every day by 0.2 mg/kg, given every 12 hours, until a maximum single dose of 1 mg/kg is reached. If the ductus remains still open, dosing interval is reduced to 8 hours so that the maximum dose is 3 mg/kg/day. The maximum duration of one course is 7–10 days.

Before start of therapy, plasmatic coagulation parameters, platelet count, serum creatinine and electrolytes are assessed and corrected if necessary. We do not try to achieve ductal closure by fluid restriction but reduce daily fluid intake by 30% at the onset of indomethacin therapy to avoid fluid overload and hyponatremia. Thereafter, fluid and electrolyte administration are adjusted daily according to the daily measured body weight and serum electrolytes, aiming to keep weight constant during therapy. Low serum levels of sodium are treated with additional fluid restriction. When urine output declines below 1 ml/kg/h, furosemide 0.5 to 1 mg/kg is given. Oral feeding is continued throughout the indomethacin treatment.

Effectiveness and Side Effects of Escalating High-Dose Therapy

To evaluate the effectiveness and side effects of our treatment algorithm delineated above we conducted a retrospective analysis of all patients born in our Perinatal Center at the University Hospital in Heidelberg, Germany between January 1993 and December 2002 [23]. During this period a total of 1267 preterm infants below <33 weeks of gestation were born. 167 (13%) received the diagnosis of sPDA and were treated with indomethacin. Twenty one infants were excluded because of accompanying congenital heart disease (n=9), congenital renal disease (n=4), other congenital diseases (n=8), or maternal disease (n=3). Seventeen additional infants were excluded because the available charts were incomplete. 129 of the 167 infants were included in the final analyses. None of the excluded infants underwent surgical closure of the ductus.

We successfully treated 73 (57%) of the 129 infants with a maximum single dose of 0.2 mg/kg indomethacin; 39 (30%) received >0.2 to ≤0.4 mg/kg; 8 (6%)

>0.4 to ≤0.6 mg/kg; 6 (5%) >0.6 to ≤0.8 mg/kg; and finally 3 (2%), including the 2 infants who had to undergo interventional closure of the ductus, were treated with >0.8 to ≤1 mg/kg indomethacin.

The overall closure rate was 127 out of 129 patients (98.5%). Only 2 preterms (monocygotic twins, 28 weeks of gestation) did not respond to the pharmacologic therapy, although they received a total dose of 30 mg/kg and 33 mg/kg, respectively. Both infants underwent interventional closure at the age of 1 year. It is interesting that both patients had unexpectedly low serum through levels of indomethacin (2400 μg/L and 2700 μg/L, respectively) despite the high dose given. Reopening of the ductus occurred in 14 (11%) infants studied. In these infants indomethacin therapy was restarted and, when necessary, followed by increasing doses of indomethacin according to the flow diagram in Fig. 7.1. The ductus was closed successfully in all 14 infants with reopened ductus. In addition, in infants in whom indomethacin therapy had to be interrupted because of adverse effects (n=3, 1 infant because of thrombocytopenia, 1 infant with NEC grade 1, and 1 infant with gastric perforation caused by a gastric tube), later continuation of the therapy led to ductal closure in all of them.

To investigate if there are more side effects associated with the high-dose therapy we compared the 68 infants with standard-dose therapy (up to 1.5 mg/kg total dose of indomethacin) with the 61 infants who received high-dose treatment (>1.5 mg/kg total dose). There was no difference in the clinical characteristics of the two groups shown in ◘ Table 7.1. Clinical outcome is summarized in ◘ Table 7.2. The most common causes of death in both groups were refractory hypoxemia or overwhelming infections. There were no significant differences in the incidence of NEC, gastrointestinal bleeding or perforation, IVH grades 3 and 4, and periventricular leukomalacia (PVL), indicating that high doses of indomethacin did not cause an increase in morbidity and mortality. Of special interest, high-dose indomethacin did not increase the incidence of gastrointestinal perforation or NEC, which had been reported as a severe complication during indomethacin treatment [19, 28].

Analysis of renal function demonstrated a transient increase of serum creatinine during therapy, but no difference in the two groups. Two to three weeks after therapy creatinine was slightly, but not significantly, higher in the high-dose versus standard-dose group (◘ Table 7.3). The decrease in urine output monitored during therapy was similar in the standard-dose and high-dose group (◘ Table 7.3). In addition the number of infants in the high-dose

Table 7.1. Clinical data of the standard-dose group and the high-dose group

	Standard-dose group ≤1.5 mg/kg n=68	High-dose group >1.5 mg/kg n=61	Significance
Birth weight [g]*	920 (495–1900)	881 (380–1730)	n.s.
Gestational age [weeks]*	27.1 (22.4–31.9)	26.6 (23.0–31.0)	n.s.
Female, n [%]	33 (50%)	33 (54%)	n.s.
Antenatal steroids, n [%]	47 (81%)	42 (72%)	n.s.
RDS, n [%]	60 (88%)	52 (87%)	n.s.

*Median (range), RDS: respiratory distress syndrome.

Table 7.2. Clinical outcome of high-dose indomethacin treatment

	Standard-dose group ≤1.5 mg/kg n=68	High-dose group >1.5 mg/kg n=61	Odds Ratio*
Death, n [%]	8 (12%)	8 (13%)	1.13 (0.4–3.2)
NEC, n [%]	4 (6%)	2 (3%)	0.5 (0.09–2.8)
GI-perforation, n [%]	0	1 (2%)	0.76 (0.03–18.9)
IHV > grade II, n [%]	7 (10%)	8 (13%)	1.4 (0.5–4.4)
PVL, n [%]	8 (12%)	9 (15%)	1.1 (0.4–3.2)

* High-dose group with higher risk of complication if odds ratio (OR) > 1. OR given as estimate with 95% confidence interval. NEC, necrotizing enterocolitis; GI, gastrointestinal; IVH, intraventricular hemorrhage; PVL, periventricular leukomalacia.

	Standard-dose group* n=68	High-dose group* n=61	Signi-ficance
Serum creatinine [mg/dL] before therapy	1.0 ± 0.3	1.0 ± 0.3	n.s.
Serum creatinine [mg/dL] during therapy	1.3 ± 0.6	1.3 ± 0.4	n.s.
Serum creatinine [mg/dL] after therapy (2–3 weeks)	0.7 ± 0.3	0.9 ± 0.5	n.s. (p=0.13)
Urine output [mL/kg/h]	2.6 ± 1.6 (9% <1 mL/kg/h)	2.8 ± 1.6 (11% <1 mL/kg/h)	n.s.
Serum sodium [mmol/L]	135 ± 6 (37% <130 mmol/L)	133 ± 7 (38% <130 mmol/L)	n.s.
Fluid intake [mL/kg/d]	96 ± 28	108 ± 38	n.s.

◘ **Table 7.3.** Renal function

*Mean ± SD

group who had urine output below 1 ml/kg/h and required treatment with furosemide was similar to the number of infants in the standard-dose group (11% vs. 9%). Fluid intake to keep the weight stable during therapy was 96 ml/kg/d in the standard and 108 ml/kg/d in the high-dose group. Serum sodium levels were comparable in both groups with the same percentage of values below 130 mmol/L, 38% in the high-dose versus 37% in the standard-dose group, respectively.

Long-Term Follow-up

Even though our results show no increase in short-term side effects of a high-dose therapy with indomethacin, it remains unclear if those patients could develop symptoms later in life or even would show abnormal neurodevelopmental outcome. Therefore, our Neurodevelopmental Department at the University Hospital Heidelberg (J. Pietz, H. Philippi, G. Reuner) performed a long-term follow-up of these patients, in order to evaluate the frequency of internal and neurological symptoms and diseases after hospital discharge, and to measure and compare the developmental status of the standard-dose group and the high-dose group.

From the original 129 children 20 patients (16%) were dead at the time of study. Of the remaining 109 children, in 17 (16%) cases an actual address could not be identified, 11 families (10%) rejected to participate. The cohort enrolled in the follow-up study thus consisted of 81 subjects, 41 belonging to the standard-dose and 40 cases to the high-dose indomethacin group.

The initial data collection was conducted on the basis of two telephone interviews of about 30 minutes each and questionnaires sent to the families. Data collection included: the families social background, kind and frequency of acute and chronic internal diseases, specific symptoms of chronic lung disease (CLD, e.g. breathing difficulties, asthma, recurrent pneumonia), eating or swallowing problems, gastrointestinal symptoms (e.g. digestion, abdominal pain), urological and nephrological symptoms (e.g. oedema, infections), neurological and neurodevelopmental symptoms (e.g. delayed motor, mental or language milestones, sensory deficits, strabismus, seizures, infantile cerebral palsy (CP) or other motor symptoms, manifest handicaps).

Neurological dysfunction was defined by the observation of CP, significant motor coordination disorder, epilepsy or hydrocephalus. Visual dysfunction was defined by the observation of substantially reduced vision, strabismus or nystagmus.

The children's behaviour was assessed with the 10-point Conners short-form rating-scale for attention deficit disorder symptoms [25]. A separate questionnaire was provided to document duration and frequency of supportive early intervention procedures, such as physiotherapy, speech therapy and occupational therapy.

To assess the current developmental status the Vineland Adaptive Behaviour Scales (VABS), Interview Edition [26], was used. This interview-based inventory was designed to assess personal and social sufficiency and adaptive behaviour. The scales are applicable to handicapped and non-handicapped individuals. VABS is an open-answer, interview format, standardized, and norm-referenced questionnaire that assesses adaptive behaviour in four domains: communication, daily living skills, socialization, and motor skills. The VABS yields four separate standard scores for the domains and an overall standard score for adaptive functioning (M=100, SD=15). It is usually administered as a face-to-face interview with parents. In the current study it was employed as a telephone interview, which did not require any alterations in the procedure. Starting from biological age (corrected age for premature babies up to two years of age) there is an age dependent starting point. Specific entry and exit criteria determine the range of items used with the individual child. Items do not have to be administered in a specific order as long as all criteria are fulfilled.

Developmental dysfunction was defined by a subnormal score (<70 points) in the VABS total score and at least one of the VABS subscale scores and/or a Connor Scales Score above 15 points.

Whenever ambiguous or unclear information provided by the parents could not be elucidated during the phone interview, the families' pediatric practitioner was contacted.

Follow-up Results

Two infants in each group died after discharge from hospital. In the standard-dose group one of unexplained bradycardia and sudden death, and one of drowning (unrelated to the premature status). In the high-dose group one from untreatable BPD, and another from undetected late sepsis.

Clinical characteristics are summarized in ◘ Table 7.4, and were similar between the two groups. As expected, total indomethacin dose was five-fold higher in the high-dose group (5.8 mg/kg) compared to the standard-dose subgroup (1.0 mg/kg). There was a trend towards a slightly longer follow-up time range in the standard-dose group (mean 8.2 years) compared to the high-dose group (mean 6.9 years, Chi^2=2.9, p<0.01).

With regard to all important outcome parameters there was no difference between the 41 children with standard indomethacin treatment and the 40 children who received additional high-dose treatment. The rate of children with subnormal growth (height, weight, head circumference) was comparable for the two groups. 6% of the standard treatment and 7% of the high-dose treatment subgroup had signs of neurological dysfunction (◘ Table 7.5). With 4 (5%) children in each of the two subgroups infantile CP was the most frequent neurological disease. Epilepsy was found in 2 children of the standard-group and in 3 children of the high-dose group. Disturbed visual

□ Table 7.4. Clinical data and neurodevelopmental outcome of standard- and high-dose group

	Standard-dose group n=40					High-dose group n=40					Kruskal Wallis	
	mean	std	min	max		mean	std	min	max		Chi^2	p
Perinatal variables												
Birth weight [g]	959	304	520	1900		898	282	465	1570		0.90	0.34
Gestational age [weeks]	27.5	2.2	23	31		26.8	2.1	23	31		1.84	0.18
Artificial ventilation [days]	5.7	8.1	0	35		5.9	6.4	0	29		0.18	0.67
Total indomethacin dose [mg/kg]	1.0	0.2	0.4	1.5		5.8	8.1	1.7	33.2		61.3	0.0001
Follow-up outcome variables												
Follow-up time [years]	8.2	3.2	3.9	12.7		6.9	2.3	3.9	12.7		2.94	0.09
Vineland Scales of Adaptive Behavior VABS												
VABS composite score	89.9	27.3	20	146		89.0	21.3	48	136		0.14	0.71
VABS communication	86.3	21.5	20	117		86.3	18.6	53	129		0.2	0.64
VABS daily living skills	87.1	25.1	20	128		89.9	21	32	133		0.001	0.97
VABS socialization	94.8	24.3	20	145		94.1	18.4	56	127		0.18	0.67
VABS motor (below age 4 years only) n=15 standard-dose group n=16 high-dose group	99.9	33.9	12	132		100.8	19.54	60	122		0.33	0.57
Connors Parent Rating Scale short version (raw score min 0 max 30)	7.9	4.7	1	20		7.7	5.0	1	23		0.11	0.73

□ Table 7.5. Long-term follow-up

Follow-up outcome	Standard-dose group n=41		High-dose group n=40		Chi^2	
	n	%	n	%	Chi^2	p
Height <3rd percentile	8	20	6	15	0.29	0.59
Weight <3rd percentile	7	17	8	20	0.11	0.74
Head circumference <3rd percentile	8	20	5	13	0.74	0.39
Neurological dysfunction: ICP, MCD, epilepsy, hydrocephalus	5	6	6	7	0.14	0.71
Disturbed visual function: vision, nystagmus, strabismus	9	11	6	7	0.64	0.42
Behavioral-developmental dysfunction: VABS, Conners scale	11	14	9	11	0.20	0.65
Lung affection: pneumonia, asthma, BPD	10	13	10	21	2.98	0.08
Gastrointestinal symptoms, eating problems, cramping	12	15	12	15	0.01	0.94
Allergy	11	14	3	4	5.29	0.02
Interventions: physiotherapy	16	20	10	12	1.82	0.18
Interventions: occupational therapy	17	21	15	19	0.13	0.71
Interventions: speech therapy	12	15	15	19	0.61	0.43

function, most frequently strabismus, was also equally distributed among the two groups. Behavioural and developmental abnormalities were observed in both groups. The rate was 14% in the standard-dose group and 11% in the high-dose group (□ Table 7.5). Neither the VABS subscale scores nor the VABS composite score differed between the groups (□ Table 7.4). In addition, the mean Conners Parent Rating scale score was comparable for the two groups (◘ Table 7.4). Supportive therapies and early intervention was frequently applied in both groups. About every fifth child received physiotherapy, occupational therapy and speech therapy during the follow-up period. However there were no significant differences between the groups (◘ Table 7.5).

There was a trend for the observation of more lung affections in the high-dose group whereas allergies were more frequently noted in the standard-dose group. Gastrointestinal symptoms were equally distributed.

Conclusions

Our retrospective data provide substantial evidence that an escalating high-dose treatment with indomethacin up to single doses of 1mg/kg dramatically improves ductal closure rate to nearly 100%. This is of considerable clinical relevance, as it avoids surgical closure in about 20–30% of preterms, which has been shown to have significant side effects [6, 7]. We observed that standard-dose treatment in our patients led to a closure rate of 53%, which is lower than the rate of about 70% reported in most other studies [14]. However, by increasing the dose we were able to close the ductus in nearly all patients. This apparent discrepancy may be related to our treatment algorithm, which includes a rapid dose increase in case the ductus remains open early after the beginning of indomethacin treatment. Thus, in some infants the ductus may have been closed without increase of the indomethacin dose.

No increase in side effects with high-dose therapy could be demonstrated compared to the standard-dose. Mortality rate was the same and the incidences of classical morbidities of preterm babies were equal in both groups. Especially there was no difference in NEC or gastrointestinal perforation, often attributed to indomethacin treatment.

The known transient impairment of renal function caused by indomethacin was also seen in our patients but was not intensified in the high-dose group.

Most important in long-term outcome after 6–8 years no increase in neurological dysfunction and sensory impairment and no decrease of neurodevelopmental scores could be seen in the high-dose group.

Therefore, we strongly advocate the application of this strategy in preterm infants who have sPDA.

Critical Perspective Concerning High-Dose Therapy with Indomethacin

In 2008, Jegatheesan et al. published a randomized, controlled trial to determine whether higher doses of indomethacin improve the rate of PDA closure [27]. Included were all preterms below 28 weeks of gestation, a group with a high risk for developing sPDA. After two prophylactic doses with 0.1 mg/kg on day one and two of life, echocardiography was performed, and all patients in whom the ductus was still open were eligible for the study. Infants were than randomized to a low-dose group, which received three additional doses with 0.1 mg/kg/day on day three to five and a high-dose group, which received 0.2 mg/kg/day (26–27 weeks of gestation) and 0.2 or 0.5 mg/kg/day (24–25 weeks of gestation) on day three to five. The 0.2 mg/kg/day arm in the 24–25 weeks of gestation group was stopped early in the study because an interim analysis showed no effect on ductal closure rate. The study drug was given in 12-hour intervals. 105 children were enrolled.

Results are shown in ◘ Table 7.6. There was no significant increase in closure rate of the ductus arteriosus in the high-dose group (55% vs. 48%). In both groups about one third had to undergo surgical ligation. Mortality was the same in both groups (16%). Most clinical outcomes were similar in the low- and high-dose group. Only in the rate of moderate to severe ROP there was a significant increase in the high-dose group (36% vs. 15%, p=0.024).

On the basis of these results, the authors conclusion is, that this treatment strategy cannot be recommended at the moment because there is no increase of the ductal closure rate in the high-dose group and on the other hand an increase in the rate of moderate to severe ROP.

Some points of the study have to be addressed. First of all, the high-dose treatment with a maximum dose of indomethacin of 0.2–0.5 mg/kg/day is in the range of our standard-dose (5 times 0.2 mg/kg) or slightly higher. When we look at the subgroup of patients with the highest dose of 0.5 mg/kg/day (24–25 weeks of gestation) there is an increase in the closure rate from 41% to 54%, which is not significant, but a clear trend. In addition, there is some evi-

□ Table 7.6. Randomized, controlled trial with high-dose indomethacin (Jegatheesan et al. [27])

	Low-dose group n=50	High-dose group n=55	P-value
Closure rate, total	48%	55%	n. s.
Closure rate, 24–25 weeks of gestation 0.5 mg/kg/day	41% (n=27)	54% (n=24)	n. s.
Ligation	32%	36%	n. s.
Indomethacin serum concentration [ng/mL]	774 + 457	1849 + 1345	<0.001
Death	16%	16%	n. s.
Intraventricular hemorrhage > grade 2	8%	9%	n.s.
Periventricular leukomalacia	7%	12%	n.s.
Necrotizing entercolitis	20%	17%	n.s.
Chronic lung disease	62%	58%	n.s.
Moderate/severe ROP	15%	36%	0.024

dence that the indomethacin level necessary for ductal closure has to be sustained for a longer period (>72 h) for permanent closure [26, 32] than in the study of Jegatheesan et al.

A very critical point is the increase in the rate of moderate to severe ROP in the high-dose group seen in the study of Jegatheesan et al. We have no data on this topic in our study population, but in our long-term follow-up we could not demonstrate an increase in visual impairment in the high-dose group. For sure this question has to be re-evaluated very carefully.

High-Dose Therapy with Ibuprofen

Few data exist about high-dose therapy with ibuprofen. With standard dosing of 10, 5 and 5 mg/kg in 24-hour intervals a ductal closure rate of about 70% is achieved, which is the same as with the standard-dose treatment with indomethacin. With ibuprofen there seems to be a lower rate of NEC but possibly a higher rate of CLD, compared to indomethacin [14, 15]. Failure of treatment occurs in very low gestational week infants and especially with older postnatal age [29]. A pharmacokinetic study published in 2008 [30] shows an increase of ibuprofen clearance from postnatal day 1 to day 8 but not with gestational age. A relationship was shown between ibuprofen area under the curve (AUC) and PDA closure rate, and an effective threshold AUC was evidenced. Dosing schemes were proposed as a function of postnatal age, to achieve this AUC and to improve the efficacy of treatment. Preterms below 70 h of age should receive a dose of 10, 5 and 5 mg/kg as previously recommended; between 70 h and 108 h of postnatal age the dose should be 14, 7 and 7 mg/kg; neonates between 108 and 180 h should receive a minimum dose of 18, 9 and 9 mg/kg. By simulations with these doses a ductal closing rate between 80% and 98% was predicted.

Until now, no published data with high-dose ibuprofen are available. One concern is increased bilirubin toxicity with higher doses.

Table 7.7. High-dose therapy with ibuprofen (M. Schroth, Erlangen)

	Standard-dose ibuprofen	High-dose ibuprofen
Number of patients	17	14
Gestational age [weeks]	28.2	30.7
Birth weight [kg]	1.14	1.52
Start of therapy [day]	3.7	3.5
3 doses	10 (59%)	12 (86%)
> 3 doses	7 (41%)	2 (14%)
Surgical ligation	4 (24%)	0
Dose 1, 2, 3 [mg/kg]	10.9–6.4–6.4	19.2–8.6–8.6

□ Table 7.8. Side effects of high-dose therapy with ibuprofen (M. Schroth, Erlangen)

	Standard-dose ibuprofen n=17	High-dose ibuprofen n=14
Re-opening [n]	1	1
Renal failure [n]	0	0
NEC [n]	0	0
ROP (higher grade) [n]	1	1
IVH > II° [n]	2	1
BPD [n]	1	2
Death [n]	0	0

Preliminary data from a retrospective analysis, made available by Dr. Schroth from the University of Erlangen, with a high-dose treatment of 20, 10 and 10 mg/kg show an increase in ductal closure rate to 86%, compared to 59% in the standard-dose group (□ Table 7.7). After two additional doses all ducts were closed in the high-dose group whereas 4 patients (24%) in the standard-dose group had to undergo surgical ligation. No short-term side effects of the high-dose therapy could be demonstrated (□ Table 7.8). From these data there is a clear trend to a higher efficacy with higher doses of ibuprofen which has to be confirmed in larger cohorts.

Outlook

At the moment, therapy of a sPDA in the preterm with a COX inhibitor in the first week of life seems to be the treatment option of choice. With standard dosing of indomethacin and ibuprofen a closing rate of about 70% is achieved. Currently, no definite evidence-based long-term benefit of this strategy can be demonstrated. Surgical ligation seems to lead to an increase in the rate of CLD, ROP and severe neurosensory impairment at long-term follow-up and should be considered as last option in selected infants who have failed pharmacological treatment.

With an escalating high-dose treatment with indomethacin closure rate of the PDA can be increased to nearly 100% and avoids surgical ligation. Our data show no short- or long-term risk of this strategy, but the increased risk for ROP shown in the study by Jegatheesan et al. [27] has to be re-evaluated very carefully. From theoretical considerations and preliminary data shown above it seems likely that with a high-dose treatment with ibuprofen the ductal closure rate can also be increased significantly. This has to be evaluated in further studies and in addition it has to be shown that this strategy is not associated with short or long-term harm of the preterms.

References

1. The Vermont-Oxford Trials Network (1993) Very low birth weight outcomes for 1990. Investigators of the Vermont-Oxford Trials Network Database Project. Pediatrics 91: 540–545
2. Fanaroff AA, Stoll BJ, Wright LL et al. (2007) Trends in neonatal morbidity and mortality for very low birthweight infants. Am J Obstet Gynecol 196: e1–8
3. Amin SB, Handley C, Carter-Prokas O (2007) Indomethacin use for the management of patent ductus arteriosus in preterms: a web based survey of practice attitudes among neonatal fellowship program directors in the United states. Pediatr Cardiol 28: 193-200
4. Hoellering AB, Cooke L (2009) The management of patent ductus arteriosus in Australia and New Zealand. J Paediatr Child Health 45: 204–209
5. Herrman K, Bose C, Lewis K, Laughon M (2009) Spontaneous closure of the patent ductus arteriosus in very low birth weight infants following discharge from the neonatal unit. Arch Dis Child Fetal Neonatal Ed 94: F48–50
6. Kabra NS, Schmidt B, Roberts RS, Doyle LW, Papile L, Fanaroff A, and the Trial of Indomethacin Prophylaxis in Preterms (TIPP) Investigators (2007) Neurosensory impairment after surgical closure of patent ductus arteriosus in extremely low birth weight infants: results from the trial of indomethacin prophylaxis in preterms. J Pediatr 150: 229–234
7. Raval MV, Laughon MM, Bose CL, Phillips JD (2007) Patent ductus arteriosus ligation in premature infants: who really benefits, and at what costs ? J Pediatr Surg 42: 69–75
8. Ahlfors CE (2004) Effect of ibuprofen on bilirubin-albumin binding. J Pediatr 144: 386–388
9. Ohlsson A, Shah SS (2006) Ibuprofen for the prevention of patent ductus arteriosus in preterm and/or low birth weight infants. Cochrane database Syst Rev 1: CD004213
10. Clyman RI, Chorne N (2007) Patent ductus arteriosus: evidence for and against treatment. J Pediatr 150: 216–219
11. Fowlie PW, Davis PG, McGuire W (2010) Prophylactic intravenous indomethacin for preventing mortality and morbidity in preterm infants. Cochrane Database Syst Rev 7: CD000174

12. Ment LR, Oh W, Ehrenkranz RA et al. (1994) Low dose indomethacin and prevention of intraventricular hemorrhage: a multicenter randomized trial. Pediatrics 93: 543–550

13. Chorne N, Jegatheesan P, Lin E, Shi R, Clyman RI (2007) Risk factors for persistent ductus arteriosus patency during indomethacin treatment. J Pediatr 151: 629–634

14. Jones LJ, Craven PD, Attia J et al. (2010) Network meta-analyses of indomethacin versus ibuprofen versus placebo for PDA in preterm infants. Arch Dis Child Fetal Neonatal Ed (published online September 27)

15. Ohlsson A, Walia R, Shah SS (2010) Ibuprofen for the treatment of patent ductus arteriosus in preterm and/or low birth weight infants. Cochrane database Syst Rev 4: CD003481

16. Gal P, Ransom JL, Weaver RL, Schall S, Wyble LE, Carlos RQ et al. (1991) Indomethacin pharmacokinetics in neonates: the value of volume of distribution as a marker of permanent patent ductus arteriosus closure. The Drug Monit 13: 42–45

17. Seyberth HW, Knapp G, Wolf D, Ulmer HE (1983) Introduction of plasma indomethacin level monitoring and evaluation of an effective threshold level in very low birth weight infants with symptomatic patent ductus arteriosus. Eur J Pediatr 141: 71–76

18. Yeh TF, Achanti B, Jain R, Patel H, Pildes RS (1989) Indomethacin therapy in premature infants with PDA – determination of therapeutic plasma levels. Dev Pharmacol Ther 12: 169–178

19. Schuster V, von Stockhausen HB, Seyberth HW (1990) Effects of highly overdosed indomethacin in apreterm infant with symptomatic patent ductus arteriosus. Eur J Pediatr 149: 651–653

20. Narayanan M, Schlueter M, Clyman RI (1999) Incidence and outcome of a 10-fold indomethacin overdose in premature infants. J Pediatr 135: 105–107

21. Seyberth HW, Königer SJ, Rascher W, Kühl G, Schweer H (1987) Role of prostaglandins in hyperprostaglandin E syndrome and in selected renal tubular disorders. Pediatr Nephrol 1: 491–497

22. Jackson JK, Abdel-Rahman SM, Reavey D, Leeks S, Garg U, Hall RT (2000) Use of indomethacin serum concentration in predicting effectiveness of dosing for symptomatic patent ductus arteriosus [abstract]. Hot Topics in Neonatology. Washington DC, p 352

23. Sperandio M, Beedgen B, Feneberg R, Huppertz C, Brüssau J, Pöschl J et al. (2005) Effectiveness and side effects of an escalating, stepwise approach to indomethacin treatment for symptomatic patent ductus arteriosus in premature infants below 33 weeks of gestation. Pediatrics 116: 1361–1366

24. Fujii AM, Brown E, Mirochnick M, O`Brien S, Kaufman G (2002) Neonatal necrotizing enterocolitis with intestinal perforation in extremely premature infants receiving early indomethacin treatment for patent ductus arteriosus. J Perinatol 22: 535–540

25. Conners CK (1973) Rating scales for use in drug studies with children. Psychopharmacol Bull (special issue – Pharmacotherapy of Children): 24–29

26. Sparrow SS, Balla DA, Ciccetti DV (1984) Vineland Adaptive Behavior Scales. Interview Edition. AGS American Guidance Service Inc., Circle Pines, Minnesota, USA

27. Jegatheesan P, Ianus V, Buchh B, Yoon G, Clyman R et al. (2008) Increased indomethacin dosing for persistent patent ductus arteriosus in preterm infants: a multicenter, randomized, controlled trial. J Pediatr 153: 183–189
28. Quinn D, Cooper B, Clyman RI (2002) Factors associated with permanent closure of the ductus arteriosus: a role for prolonged indomethacin therapy. Pediatrics 110: e10
29. Desfrere L, Zohar, S, Morville P, Treluyer J.M. et al. (2005) Dose-finding study of ibuprofen in patent ductus arteriosus using the continual reassessment method. J Clin Pharm Ther 30: 121–132
30. Hirt D, Van Overmeire B, Treluyer JM, Urien S et al. (2008) An optimized ibuprofen dosing scheme for preterm neonates with patent ductus arteriosus, based on a population pharmacokinetic and pharmacodynamic study. Br J Clin Pharmacol 65: 629–636

8

Risks and Benefits of Aggressive and Conservative Approaches to the Management of the Patent Ductus Arteriosus in Premature Infants

S. Aliaga, M.M. Laughon

Introduction

During fetal life, the ductus arteriosus (DA) connects the pulmonary artery to the aorta and provides a channel through which the majority of pulmonary blood flow is shunted into the systemic circulation. Persistent patency of the DA during the first few days after birth might represent a normal physiologic adaptation by allowing shunting from pulmonary to systemic circulation as the left ventricle adapts to its role as the dominant pumping chamber. However, in the vast majority of infants, the DA closes by three days of life [1]. In some infants, especially preterm infants with lung disease, there is a delayed closure of the DA [2]. Approximately 65% of infants born at less than 28 weeks' gestation will have a diagnosis of a patent ductus arteriosus (PDA) at some time during the early neonatal period [3].

Premature infants who have a diagnosis of a PDA are more likely to develop bronchopulmonary dysplasia (BPD), and a PDA is associated with necrotizing enterocolitis (NEC). Although a cause and effect relationship between the diagnosis of a PDA and mortality or morbidities of prematurity has not been established, most neonatologists attempt to close a PDA if it is considered "symptomatic", usually based on a combination of clinical signs and an echocardiogram. Medical treatment of a PDA with a prostaglandin inhibitor (e.g., indomethacin or ibuprofen), or surgical ligation if medical treatment fails, has become a "standard of care" in many neonatal units [4]. However, there is little evidence to suggest that treatment of a PDA reduces the incidence of death, BPD, NEC, or other morbidities. Treatment with indomethacin, ibuprofen, and/or surgical ligation is associated with significant adverse effects such as intestinal perforation [5] and vocal cord paralysis [6], respectively. Without a precise understanding of the benefits of closure of a symptomatic PDA and the risks of therapies, clinicians cannot make informed decisions about treatment for this common problem. It is possible that elective closure of the DA causes significant morbidity without benefit.

In this chapter, we will review the evidence of the association between a PDA and morbidities of prematurity, risks and benefits of medical and surgical therapies of a PDA, the current variation in treatment approaches among centres, and outline our rationale that current evidence does not support an aggressive approach to treatment of a PDA.

PDA and Clinical Outcomes

A diagnosis of a PDA has been traditionally associated with the development of BPD and NEC, and more recently surgical ligation has been associated with the development of neurodevelopmental impairment. In this section, we will review the association between a PDA and clinical outcomes, first examining the pathophysiologic consequences of a PDA, next by examining epidemiological associations between PDA and the morbidity of interest, and finally by examining results from randomized, controlled trials (RCTs).

PDA and Bronchopulmonary Dysplasia

A PDA is thought to decrease lung compliance via an increase in pulmonary circulation and resultant increased lung water. Some evidence in humans is suggested by a small longitudinal study examining lung compliance. In 9 premature infants receiving mechanical ventilation diagnosed with a PDA, closure improved dynamic compliance and increased tidal volume [7]. If clinicians increased ventilator settings to address the poor compliance, this finding might explain how a PDA could increase the risk of BPD.

In population-based or centre-based cohorts of premature infants, a PDA has been associated with the outcome of BPD. Rojas et al examined a cohort of 119 infants weighing less than 1000 g in a single centre and demonstrated that the odds ratio (OR) for the development of BPD, defined by the need for oxygen therapy at 28 days or longer, was 6.2 for infants with a PDA and 48.3 when PDA and sepsis occurred simultaneously [8]. In a large, prospective, population-based study of 1460 infants in North Carolina, PDA emerged as a risk factor for BPD with an OR of 1.9 [9].

Meta-analyses of RCTs suggest no change in the incidence of BPD or other morbidities following treatment [10, 11]. The Cochrane Database of Systematic Reviews currently includes two meta-analyses of the efficacy of indomethacin in the prevention or treatment of the PDA. The first review identified 19 trials designed to determine the benefits of prophylactic indomethacin. These studies enrolled infants without evidence of a PDA who were at risk of having persistent patency of the DA. The authors conclude that prophylactic indomethacin reduces the incidence of symptomatic PDA (sPDA), subsequent ligation, and the incidence of intraventricular hemorrhage (IVH). However, the meta-analysis did not show an effect on BPD, mortality, or death or neurodevelopmental disability [11].

The second review identified three trials, with a total of 97 infants, which were designed to determine the benefits of treating infants with an asymptomatic PDA with indomethacin. These studies enrolled infants with echocardiographic evidence of a PDA who did not have a left-to-right shunt of sufficient magnitude to cause symptoms. Using indomethacin in these infants decreased the incidence of sPDA and the duration of treatment with supplemental oxygen [10].

However, no change in the incidence of BPD, retinopathy of prematurity (ROP), length of ventilation, or mortality was observed following treatment. Long-term outcomes such as neurodevelopmental impairment were not reported in these trials.

There is no Cochrane Review for the treatment of a sPDA. However, three trials compared indomethacin versus placebo for the treatment of a sPDA (Gersony [12], the National Collaborative study: two of the 3 study groups, the third underwent ligation, Merritt [13], and Yeh [14]). If published data from studies on treatment of sPDA is pooled then there is no evidence of benefit for mortality (typical RR 0.93, 95% CI 0.56–1.54) or NEC (typical RR 1.11, 95% CI 0.44–2.8) and a significant increase in the risk of BPD (typical RR 1.43, 95% CI 1.05–1.96).

The largest RCT investigating the benefits of indomethacin therapy in premature infants was the Trial of Indomethacin Prophylaxis in Preterm Infants (TIPP Trial) [15]. This trial randomized 1202 infants with birth weights of 500 to 999 g to receive indomethacin or placebo. In addition to neurodevelopmental outcome (see below), the study reported morbidities during the initial hospitalization. Administration of indomethacin was associated with a lower incidence of PDA, subsequent medical treatment of the PDA, and subsequent PDA ligation, but there was no difference in the incidence of BDP or other morbidities potentially associated with a PDA (e.g. NEC, feeding intolerance, or ROP). The best estimate for the effect of prophylactic indomethacin on the development of BDP was 1.2, and the 95% confidence interval 0.9–1.5, suggesting that the use of prophylactic indomethacin is just as likely to have had a 10% reduction as a 50% increase in BDP. Indomethacin treatment was allowed in 46% of the control group, thus limiting the generalizability of the results. Similarly, off-study treatment limits the ability to draw conclusions about adverse effects of indomethacin.

There are a number of problems with the RCTs of indomethacin. The primary endpoint of the majority of these studies was not to determine whether closure improved outcomes because clinicians assumed that closure was beneficial. Thus, the benefits of closure of a PDA with the goal of reducing BPD or other morbidities have not been demonstrated. In addition, the percentage of "crossover" in infants assigned to the placebo group ranged from 65% to 85% [16]. The off-study use of indomethacin was permitted because clinicians assumed that the PDA was pathologic and, if left untreated, would contribute to morbidity. The effect of this study design was high rates of off-study treatment. Therefore, the ability to draw conclusions about benefit is dramatically compromised.

In conclusion, the diagnosis of a PDA is associated with the short-term endpoint of a decrease in lung compliance, and epidemiologic studies confirm the association between a diagnosis of a PDA and BPD. However, RCTs and meta-analyses of RCTs of indomethacin, although demonstrating a decrease in the diagnosis of PDA and an increase in closure of the PDA in the treatment groups, do not demonstrate a subsequent reduction in BPD. Clinicians should not choose to administer a COX inhibitor with the goal of reducing BPD.

PDA and Necrotizing Enterocolitis

NEC is a potentially devastating disease affecting preterm infants, and some believe that a PDA might contribute to this disease. A PDA is thought to decrease blood flow to the intestines via a "steal syndrome" because of an increase in pulmonary circulation. This might result in decreased oxygen delivery, subsequent intestinal damage and stasis, feeding intolerance, and finally NEC.

There is some evidence – most often by using ultrasonography to measure blood flow – that a PDA might contribute to the pathophysiology of NEC. In one study, preterm infants with a hemodynamically significant PDA had higher left ventricular output and preserved cerebral blood flow, but decreased flow in the celiac, mesenteric, and renal arteries [17]. In another, preterm infants with a sPDA had absent mesenteric end diastolic forward blood flow, and in some retrograde diastolic blood flow was noted; these findings were absent in the comparison group, those infants without a symptomatic PDA [18]. In the infants with a PDA, mesenteric blood flow improved after treatment with indomethacin and subsequent ductal closure.

Epidemiologic studies generally support the association of a diagnosis of a PDA and NEC (or intestinal perforation). Sharma et al. [19] prospectively studied 992 preterm neonates and found increased odds of intestinal perforation, but not of NEC, with early administration of indomethacin for IVH prophylaxis, but not among infants treated for a PDA later in their hospitalization. In addition, these same authors demonstrated lower odds of NEC with late (>12–24 h of life) postnatal exposure to indomethacin, suggesting a protective effect of ductal closure on the risk of NEC. In 15,072 neonates with NEC or intestinal perforation in the Pediatrix Clinical Data Warehouse, indomethacin use combined with post-natal steroids during the first week of life was associated with an increased risk of NEC [20]. In a population based study in Israel, Dollberg et al. [21] found among 6146 infants of 24 to 34 weeks' gestation an independent association between PDA and NEC with an OR of 1.85. However, since treatment with indomethacin did not appear to reduce the risk of NEC, the authors speculate that the diagnosis of PDA is a non-modifiable risk factor for NEC.

The Cochrane meta-analyses of RCTs of prophylactic indomethacin (including the TIPP trial [15]) suggest no difference in the incidence of NEC between infants exposed to indomethacin versus those in the control group [10, 11]. However, these RCTs have the same problems as mentioned above: a high crossover rate and a primary outcome of closure of the PDA, not decreasing the incidence of NEC.

In conclusion, some physiologic studies support the notion that a diagnosis of PDA is associated with decreased mesenteric blood flow and that treatment with indomethacin returns those blood flows to near normal. Epidemiologic studies demonstrate that a PDA is associated with NEC, but might be a non-modifiable risk factor. RCTs and meta-analysis of RCTs of indomethacin demonstrate no difference in NEC between infants exposed versus those not exposed to indomethacin, although there was a high percentage of crossover and the studies were not designed to assess NEC as a primary endpoint. Clinicians should not choose to administer a COX inhibitor with the goal of reducing NEC.

PDA and Neurodevelopmental Impairment

The presence of neurodevelopmental impairment in preterm infants is perhaps the most important long-term clinical outcome of premature birth, aside from death. A diagnosis of a PDA might affect neurodevelopmental impairment through one of two mechanisms. A PDA might have a direct adverse effect on cerebral blood flow because a PDA has been associated with shunting through the pulmonary vasculature and reduced blood flow to post-ductal organs. A second mechanism might be through avoiding morbidities of prematurity associated with neurodevelopmental impairment, most notably IVH, BPD, and NEC [22–24], if closure of the PDA reduces the incidence of those morbidities.

Cerebral blood flow, and potentially oxygen delivery, might be impaired with a PDA. The thought is that this might lead to inadequate tissue delivery of oxygen, brain ischemia and damage, an increase in inflammatory mediators, and increased neurodevelopmental impairment under these circumstances. Some evidence for this hypothesis exists in humans. Several studies using ultrasonography measuring different parameters of cerebral blood flow in preterm infants with and without a PDA have found reduced cerebral blood flow velocity in the presence of a PDA [25–27], although not all studies support these findings [28]. Reduced cerebral oxygen saturation in the setting of a PDA has also been described using near-infrared spectroscopy [29, 30].

Treatment of a PDA with the goal of closure might reduce morbidities of prematurity, and thus decrease neurodevelopmental impairment. Prophylactic indomethacin clearly reduces the risk of severe IVH [11, 31]. Despite this finding pooled results from RCTs suggest no difference in neurodevelopmental outcomes after prophylactic indomethacin or medical closure of the PDA [11, 31]. The reduction in severe IVH after prophylactic indomethacin does not improve neurodevelopmental outcome [15]. Although infants exposed to indomethacin had a lower incidence of PDA and PDA ligation, and thus had less exposure to the hemodynamic effects of a PDA, white matter injury as seen on cranial ultrasound was similar between those exposed and not exposed to indomethacin [15]. One possibility is that the majority of infants who did not develop severe IVH and were exposed to indomethacin experienced a small degree of harm.

The association of a PDA with other morbidities of preterm birth, such as BPD and NEC, is a complex pathway in the development of neurodevelopmental impairment in the setting of a PDA. Infants with a PDA are generally smaller and less mature than those without a PDA, which are also risk factors for poor neurodevelopment. Regardless, as the incidence of BPD and NEC are not decreased in the meta-analyses, it seems unlikely that treatment of a PDA would improve neurodevelopmental outcomes through those mechanisms.

In conclusion, evidence that a PDA is associated with decreased cerebral blood flow is mixed. RCTs have demonstrated that indomethacin reduces IVH, sPDA, and PDA ligation but does not improve neurodevelopmental outcomes. However, these RCTs were not designed to assess neurodevelopmental impairment as a primary endpoint. Clinicians should not choose to administer a COX inhibitor with the goal of improving neurodevelopmental impairment.

Other systematic reviews

Two other systematic reviews have been published which examined numerous outcomes after treatments designed to prevent or close the PDA. The first examined therapies designed to close a symptomatic PDA, and grouped together ligation, intravenous indomethacin, and enteral administration of indomethacin. The author found that the only statistically significant benefit was a decreased risk of PDA (RR 0.32, 95% CI 0.23–0.44); there was no difference in NEC, ROP, BPD, or mortality [16]. The second exhaustively examined all therapies designed to close the PDA and included IV/PO indomethacin, IV/PO ibuprofen, and ligation, both prophylactically and for asymptomatic and symptomatic PDA, and found no benefit for treatment other than ductal closure [31].

Risks of Treatment

All therapies used in medicine are associated with risks and benefits. Thus far, we have examined the potential benefits of treatment of a PDA, and in this section we will review the potential risks of treatment of a PDA, including medical and surgical therapy. If the benefit of a therapeutic is minimal or none then any risks should prompt clinicians to avoid the medication. However, if the benefit is high (e.g., survival), even with high risk (e.g., immune suppression for children with oncologic conditions), then clinicians might use the medications. The balance of the benefits must outweigh the risks. As Dr. Daniel K. Benjamin Jr. wrote recently: "All drugs cause harm to at least a small proportion of children who receive them. Some drugs reduce or cure disease in children, and very few drugs benefit more children than are harmed by their use" [32].

Indomethacin

Indomethacin is associated with potentially hazardous short-term pharmaco-logic effects including altered platelet function and decreased cerebral [33, 34], mesenteric and renal blood flow [35]. Indomethacin use has also been associated with intestinal perforation [36–38] and NEC [39], potentially lethal conditions associated with morbidities such as multiple surgeries and short gut syndrome. A multi-centre trial of hydrocortisone to treat adrenal insufficiency to prevent bronchopulmonary dysplasia demonstrated an association between the combination of post-natal steroids and indomethacin and intestinal perforations [40]. Indeed, this finding led to early closure of the trial. Results from studies on the association between indomethacin exposure and NEC or intestinal perforation need to be interpreted with the consideration that the clinical diagnosis of NEC and spontaneous intestinal perforation is challenging and can lead to misdiagnosis in favour of either condition.

One theoretical risk for humans is long-term renal injury. Indomethacin is known to cause transient renal failure in premature infants [41]; however, there is little evidence to determine the potential for long-term renal consequences. In a neonatal rat model, Kent et al. found changes in glomerular and tubular structure after prenatal and postnatal exposure to indomethacin and ibuprofen [42]. Injury due to exposure to these medications could possibly lead to decreased numbers of nephrons and subsequent chronic renal effects.

Ibuprofen

Ibuprofen is used as an alternative to indomethacin for treatment of a PDA, primarily due to fewer clinically apparent renal side effects. Ibuprofen received

FDA approval in 2006 in the United States for use in treatment of clinically significant PDAs. A multicenter study in France [43] evaluated renal function at baseline and at one month of age in premature infants meeting echocardiographic criteria for treatment with ibuprofen at 2 days of age. These results were compared to controls not meeting echocardiographic criteria for treatment with ibuprofen. The glomerular filtration rate was significantly lower in those treated with ibuprofen, and this finding was still present at one month of age.

A recent Cochrane review [44] found that compared to indomethacin, ibuprofen appears to be as effective in closing the PDA, and reduces the risk of NEC (RR=0.68, 95% CI 0.47–0.99) and the incidence of transient renal insufficiency. No additional benefits have been found, and a recent meta-analysis found an increased risk of BPD in infants exposed to ibuprofen for treatment of a PDA [45].

Surgical Ligation

Surgical ligation of the PDA is a treatment option when medical therapy has failed to lead to closure of the PDA; it has also been used as an alternative to early medical prophylactic closure. The only trial where ligation of the PDA has demonstrated some benefit enrolled 87 premature infants and compared prophylactic ductal ligation (<24 hours of life) to standard care without the use of medical therapy for closure. In this trial, there was a statistical difference in the development of NEC, with an advantage for the infants who received ligation [46]. However, the diagnosis of NEC is challenging and subject to interpretation of radiographs. Mortality was not different between groups, and a subsequent reexamination of the data demonstrates an increase risk in the development of BPD at 36 weeks [47]. Current practice does not include routine prophylactic surgical ligation.

More recently, increasing data about the risks associated with PDA ligation are accumulating. Surgical ligation of the ductus is associated with significant morbidities, including vocal cord paralysis, feeding difficulties, and growth failure [6]; increased risk of BPD and ROP [48]; scoliosis [49]; and neurodevelopmental impairment [48, 50]. In addition, in a longitudinal study design, Jhaveri et al. demonstrated that a "less aggressive" approach, reserving PDA ligation for infants with "respiratory failure", was associated with a decrease in the incidence of NEC [51]. Since infants who receive a PDA ligation are usually smaller and more immature than their peers [52], it is not clear whether PDA ligation is causative of poor long-term outcome or merely a marker of disease severity [48]. A recent study using near-infrared spectroscopy during PDA ligation in preterm infants showed decreased cerebral oxygen saturation in 13 out of 20 infants undergoing surgery [30]. The lack of evidence of benefit from surgical closure of the DA, combined with the risk of surgical morbidities and the potential for worse outcomes after ligation (increased BDP, ROP, and neurodevelopmental impairment) do not support the use of this treatment option for the routine management of a PDA.

Center (Centre) Variation in Treatment of the PDA

Given that the risks and benefits of therapies for closure are uncertain, there is no clear course of action for providers. This medical uncertainty is reflected in wide practice variation in both medical and surgical therapies. Medical therapies for a PDA vary widely depending on the centre. Providers from units operated by Pediatrix Medical Group, Inc exhibit a wide practice variation, from 0–100% of infants with a diagnosis of a PDA receiving indomethacin therapy, depending on the centre [52]. Rates of PDA ligation vary dramatically among centres, and low rates do not appear to adversely affect outcomes. To the contrary, low rates of ligation are associated with potential benefit. For example, in the TIPP Trial, rates of ligation among centres ranged from 0 to greater than 20% [3]. Centres that had higher rates of ligation had a higher risk of death or neurodevelopmental impairment. After adjustment for antenatal steroid use, gestational age at birth, sex, multiple births, and maternal education, the association between rates of ligation and outcomes was reduced, suggesting that differences in the population at the centre contributed to a portion of the observed variability in outcomes.

Two different centre approaches illustrate the wide difference in management styles of a PDA, with similar outcomes. An aggressive treatment is reported by a single centre from the University of California at San Francisco [4]. In a longitudinal study design, the authors examined an "aggressive" treatment from 1999–2004, consisting of an echocardiogram on postnatal day 2–3, 3 doses of indomethacin (6 doses if the ductus remained patent), followed by ligation of all PDAs; compared to a "conservative" treatment from 2005–2008 consisting of an echocardiogram on postnatal day 2–3, 3 doses of indomethacin (6 doses if the ductus remains patent), followed by ligation only if "cardiopulmonary compromise" was present. All infants received indomethacin for prophylactic closure of the ductus. In the aggressive arm 100% of PDAs that persisted after medical therapies were subsequently ligated. In the conservative treatment period 72% were ligated. The conservative approach was associated with decreased rates of duct ligation (72% vs. 100%; p<0.05). Even though infants subjected to this approach were exposed to larger PDA shunts for longer durations, the rates of BPD, sepsis, ROP, neurologic injury, and death were lower than with the aggressive treatment approach. The overall rate of NEC was significantly lower in the "conservative" treatment period compared with the "aggressive" treatment period. Thus, a "conservative approach" to ligation is not harmful and might be beneficial.

An even more conservative treatment was reported by a group from Belgium [51]. The authors examined an "aggressive" approach from 1999–2004 which included an echocardiogram on postnatal day 2 or 3 and, if a PDA was found, fluid restriction and adjusting ventilation. Indomethacin or ibuprofen treatment (either prophylactic or treatment) was not used and surgical ligation was performed if the infant developed cardiopulmonary compromise. The "conservative" approach from 2005–2006 included an echocardiogram on postnatal day 2 or 3, and if a PDA was found, fluid restriction and adjusting ventilation. There was no treatment with indomethacin or ibuprofen and no PDA ligations were perfomed. There was little difference in common morbidities of prematurity between the aggressive and conservative groups, and both eras had similar rates as the Vermont Oxford Network. Rates of NEC, IVH, BPD, and death were 0, 7, 8, and 13% in the aggressive group and 0, 2, 7, and 12% in the conservative group. Thus, a conservative approach to medical therapy results in outcomes that are similar to the outcome in centres where medical therapy is common, and avoidance of ligation is not harmful.

Conclusion

Despite the widely held belief among neonatologists that a PDA contributes to the pathogenesis of BPD and that closure of a PDA reduces the incidence of BPD or other morbidities [53], there have been no randomized, controlled trials that have been designed to answer this question in the modern era. The use of these therapies is considered "standard of care" because benefits of closure of the PDA (i.e., association with BPD or NEC) might outweigh the risks of these therapies. Evidence for the use of medical and surgical treatment for closure of the PDA in preterm infants does not show clear benefit and in many instances proven harm, particularly known consequences of surgical ligation. Treatment with indomethacin is associated with significant risks, such as intestinal perforation, and these risks are serious enough to potentially outweigh the benefits. The net result may be that one of the most widely used therapies in neonatal medicine exposes infants to substantial harm without compensatory benefit.

Unfortunately, no trial has been performed to properly evaluate the benefits relative to the risks associated with aggressive (treatment of a symptomatic PDA) versus conservative (treatment in the setting of congestive heart failure) management strategies to close the PDA. Therefore, until randomized, controlled trials determine the risks and benefits of aggressive versus conservative treatments of a PDA in preterm infants, the best available evidence suggests that a conservative approach is best for infants.

References

1. Gentile R, Stevenson G, Dooley T, Franklin D, Kawabori I, Pearlman A (1981) Pulsed Doppler echocardiographic determination of time of ductal closure in normal newborn infants. J Pediatr 98: 443–448
2. Clyman R, Narayanan M (2000) Patent ductus arteriosus: a physiologic basis for current treatment practices. WB Saunders, Philadelphia
3. Costeloe K, Hennessy E, Gibson AT, Marlow N, Wilkinson AR (2000) The EPICure study: outcomes to discharge from hospital for infants born at the threshold of viability. Pediatrics 106: 659–671
4. Jhaveri N, Moon-Grady A, Clyman RI (2010) Early surgical ligation versus a conservative approach for management of patent ductus arteriosus that fails to close after indomethacin treatment. J Pediatr 157: 381–387
5. Gordon PV, Attridge JT (2009) Understanding clinical literature relevant to spontaneous intestinal perforations. Am J Perinatol 26: 309–316
6. Benjamin JR, Smith PB, Cotten CM, Jaggers J, Goldstein RF, Malcolm WF (2010) Long-term morbidities associated with vocal cord paralysis after surgical closure of a patent ductus arteriosus in extremely low birth weight infants. J Perinatol 30: 408–413
7. Stefano JL, Abbasi S, Pearlman SA, Spear ML, Esterly KL, Bhutani VK (1991) Closure of the ductus arteriosus with indomethacin in ventilated neonates with respiratory distress syndrome. Effects of pulmonary compliance and ventilation. Am Rev Respir Dis 143: 236–239

8. Rojas MA, Gonzalez A, Bancalari E, Claure N, Poole C, Silva-Neto G (1995) Changing trends in the epidemiology and pathogenesis of neonatal chronic lung disease. J Pediatr 126: 605–610
9. Marshall DD, Kotelchuck M, Young TE, Bose CL, Kruyer L, O'Shea TM (1999) Risk factors for chronic lung disease in the surfactant era: a North Carolina population-based study of very low birth weight infants. North Carolina Neonatologists Association. Pediatrics 104: 1345–1350
10. Cooke L, Steer P, Woodgate P (2003) Indomethacin for asymptomatic patent ductus arteriosus in preterm infants. Cochrane Database Syst Rev CD003745
11. Fowlie PW, Davis PG, McGuire W (2010) Prophylactic intravenous indomethacin for preventing mortality and morbidity in preterm infants. Cochrane Database Syst Rev CD000174
12. Gersony WM, Peckham GJ, Ellison RC, Miettinen OS, Nadas AS (1983) Effects of indomethacin in premature infants with patent ductus arteriosus: results of a national collaborative study. J Pediatr 102: 895–906
13. Merritt TA, Harris JP, Roghmann K et al. (1981) Early closure of the patent ductus arteriosus in very low-birth-weight infants: a controlled trial. J Pediatr 99: 281–286
14. Yeh TF, Luken JA, Thalji A, Raval D, Carr I, Pildes RS (1981) Intravenous indomethacin therapy in premature infants with persistent ductus arteriosus--a double-blind controlled study. J Pediatr 98: 137–145
15. Schmidt B, Davis P, Moddemann D et al. (2001) Long-term effects of indomethacin prophylaxis in extremely-low-birth-weight infants. N Engl J Med 344: 1966–1972
16. Knight DB (2001) The treatment of patent ductus arteriosus in preterm infants. A review and overview of randomized trials. Semin Neonatol 6: 63–73
17. Shimada S, Kasai T, Konishi M, Fujiwara T (1994) Effects of patent ductus arteriosus on left ventricular output and organ blood flows in preterm infants with respiratory distress syndrome treated with surfactant. J Pediatr 125: 270–277
18. Coombs RC, Morgan ME, Durbin GM, Booth IW, McNeish AS (1990) Gut blood flow velocities in the newborn: effects of patent ductus arteriosus and parenteral indomethacin. Arch Dis Child 65: 1067–1071
19. Sharma R, Hudak ML, Tepas JJ 3rd et al. (2010) Prenatal or postnatal indomethacin exposure and neonatal gut injury associated with isolated intestinal perforation and necrotizing enterocolitis. J Perinatol 30: 786–793
20. Guthrie SO, Gordon PV, Thomas V, Thorp JA, Peabody J, Clark RH (2003) Necrotizing enterocolitis among neonates in the United States. J Perinatol 23: 278–225
21. Dollberg S, Lusky A, Reichman B (2005) Patent ductus arteriosus, indomethacin and necrotizing enterocolitis in very low birth weight infants: a population-based study. J Pediatr Gastroenterol Nutr 40: 184–188
22. Hintz SR, Kendrick DE, Stoll BJ et al. (2005) Neurodevelopmental and growth outcomes of extremely low birth weight infants after necrotizing enterocolitis. Pediatrics 115: 696–703
23. Laughon M, O'Shea MT, Allred EN et al. (2009) Chronic lung disease and developmental delay at 2 years of age in children born before 28 weeks' gestation. Pediatrics 124: 637–648

24. Van Marter LJ, Kuban KC, Allred E et al. (2011) Does bronchopulmonary dysplasia contribute to the occurrence of cerebral palsy among infants born before 28 weeks of gestation? Arch Dis Child Fetal Neonatal Ed 96: F20–29

25. Weir FJ, Ohlsson A, Myhr TL, Fong K, Ryan ML (1999) A patent ductus arteriosus is associated with reduced middle cerebral artery blood flow velocity. Eur J Pediatr 158: 484–487

26. Lipman B, Serwer GA, Brazy JE (1982) Abnormal cerebral hemodynamics in preterm infants with patent ductus arteriosus. Pediatrics 69: 778–781

27. Perlman JM, Hill A, Volpe JJ (1981) The effect of patent ductus arteriosus on flow velocity in the anterior cerebral arteries: ductal steal in the premature newborn infant. J Pediatr 99: 767–771

28. Shimada S, Kasai T, Hoshi A, Murata A, Chida S (2003) Cardiocirculatory effects of patent ductus arteriosus in extremely low-birth-weight infants with respiratory distress syndrome. Pediatr Int 45: 255–262

29. Lemmers PM, Toet MC, van Bel F (2008) Impact of patent ductus arteriosus and subsequent therapy with indomethacin on cerebral oxygenation in preterm infants. Pediatrics 121: 142–147

30. Lemmers PM, Molenschot MC, Evens J, Toet MC, van Bel F (2010) Is cerebral oxygen supply compromised in preterm infants undergoing surgical closure for patent ductus arteriosus? Arch Dis Child Fetal Neonatal Ed 95: F429–434

31. Benitz W (2010) Treatment of persistent patent ductus arteriosus in preterm infants: time to accept the null hypothesis? J Perinatol 30: 241–252

32. Benjamin DK Jr (2008) First, do no harm. Pediatrics 121: 831–832

33. Lundell BP, Sonesson SE, Cotton RB (1986) Ductus closure in preterm infants. Effects on cerebral hemodynamics. Acta Paediatr Scand Suppl 329: 140–147

34. Edwards AD, Wyatt JS, Richardson C et al. (1990) Effects of indomethacin on cerebral haemodynamics in very preterm infants. Lancet 335: 1491–1495

35. Pezzati M, Vangi V, Biagiotti R, Bertini G, Cianciulli D, Rubaltelli FF (1999) Effects of indomethacin and ibuprofen on mesenteric and renal blood flow in preterm infants with patent ductus arteriosus. J Pediatr 135: 733–738

36. Nagaraj HS, Sandhu AS, Cook LN, Buchino JJ, Groff DB (1981) Gastrointestinal perforation following indomethacin therapy in very low birth weight infants. J Pediatr Surg 16: 1003–1007

37. Kuhl G, Wille L, Bolkenius M, Seyberth HW (1985) Intestinal perforation associated with indomethacin treatment in premature infants. Eur J Pediatr 143: 213–216

38. Aschner JL, Deluga KS, Metlay LA, Emmens RW, Hendricks-Munoz KD (1988) Spontaneous focal gastrointestinal perforation in very low birth weight infants. J Pediatr 113: 364–367

39. Fujii AM, Brown E, Mirochnick M, O'Brien S, Kaufman G (2002) Neonatal necrotizing enterocolitis with intestinal perforation in extremely premature infants receiving early indomethacin treatment for patent ductus arteriosus. J Perinatol 22: 535–540

40. Watterberg KL, Gerdes JS, Cole CH et al. (2004) Prophylaxis of early adrenal insufficiency to prevent bronchopulmonary dysplasia: a multicenter trial. Pediatrics 114: 1649–1657

41. Srinivasjois RM, Nathan EA, Doherty DA, Patole SK (2006) Renal impairment associated with indomethacin treatment for patent ductus arteriosus in extremely preterm neonates – is postnatal age at start of treatment important? J Matern Fetal Neonatal Med 19: 793–799

42. Kent AL, Maxwell LE, Koina ME, Falk MC, Willenborg D, Dahlstrom JE (2007) Renal glomeruli and tubular injury following indomethacin, ibuprofen, and gentamicin exposure in a neonatal rat model. Pediatr Res 62: 307–312

43. Vieux R, Desandes R, Boubred F et al. (2010) Ibuprofen in very preterm infants impairs renal function for the first month of life. Pediatr Nephrol 25: 267–274

44. Ohlsson A, Walia R, Shah SS (2010) Ibuprofen for the treatment of patent ductus arteriosus in preterm and/or low birth weight infants. Cochrane Database Syst Rev CD003481

45. Jones LJ, Craven PD, Attia J, Thakkinstian A, Wright I (2011) Network meta-analysis of indomethacin versus ibuprofen versus placebo for PDA in preterm infants. Arch Dis Child Fetal Neonatal Ed 96: F45–52

46. Cassady G, Crouse DT, Kirklin JW et al. (1989) A randomized, controlled trial of very early prophylactic ligation of the ductus arteriosus in babies who weighed 1000 g or less at birth. N Engl J Med 320: 1511–1516

47. Clyman R, Cassady G, Kirklin JK, Collins M, Philips JB 3rd (2009) The role of patent ductus arteriosus ligation in bronchopulmonary dysplasia: reexamining a randomized controlled trial. J Pediatr 154: 873–876

48. Kabra NS, Schmidt B, Roberts RS, Doyle LW, Papile L, Fanaroff A (2007) Neurosensory impairment after surgical closure of patent ductus arteriosus in extremely low birth weight infants: results from the Trial of Indomethacin Prophylaxis in Preterms. J Pediatr 150: 229–234, 34e1

49. Roclawski M, Sabiniewicz R, Potaz P et al. (2009) Scoliosis in patients with aortic coarctation and patent ductus arteriosus: does standard posterolateral thoracotomy play a role in the development of the lateral curve of the spine? Pediatr Cardiol 30: 941–945

50. Madan JC, Kendrick D, Hagadorn JI, Frantz ID 3rd (2009) Patent ductus arteriosus therapy: impact on neonatal and 18-month outcome. Pediatrics 123: 674–681

51. Vanhaesebrouck S, Zonnenberg I, Vandervoort P, Bruneel E, Van Hoestenberghe MR, Theyskens C (2007) Conservative treatment for patent ductus arteriosus in the preterm. Arch Dis Child Fetal Neonatal Ed 92: F244–247

52. Laughon M, Bose C, Clark R (2007) Treatment strategies to prevent or close a patent ductus arteriosus in preterm infants and outcomes. J Perinatol 27: 164–170

53. Amin SB, Handley C, Carter-Pokras O (2007) Indomethacin use for the management of patent ductus arteriosus in preterms: a web-based survey of practice attitudes among neonatal fellowship program directors in the United States. Pediatr Cardiol 28: 193–200

9

Missing Data for an Evidence-Based Approach to the Treatment of a Patent Ductus Arteriosus
A Small Selection of What We Do not Know Yet

A. Franz

More than 50 years after the description of persistent patency of the arterial duct in preterm infants [1], there is still or rather again controversy on the appropriate management of the patent duct despite publication of more than 75 randomized controlled trials that enrolled more than 6617 patients [2].

Evidence-based medical practice requires that clinicians make use of the best research they can find to help them in decision-making. To find this best research, clinicians have to ask questions including these elements:

- **P**atients
- **I**ntervention
- **C**ontrol/comparative intervention
- **O**utcome

In this chapter the most pressing open research questions regarding therapy of the open duct will be summarized applying this structure to both prophylactic and therapeutic interventions aiming to close the duct.

The patent duct arteriosus (PDA) is associated with numerous complications of prematurity such as bronchopulmonary dysplasia [3–5], pulmonary hemorrhage [6], necrotizing enterocolitis [7], renal impairment [7], intraventricular hemorrhage [8, 9], periventricular leukomalacia [10], cerebral palsy [11], and an increased risk of death [12, 13].

Ductal steal inappropriately decreases systemic perfusion and increases pulmonary perfusion. Based on the associations of a PDA with the complications described above and these pathophysiological considerations, it may seem appropriate to close the PDA by medical or surgical therapy as soon as possible. Particularly as there are highly efficacious interventions to close the PDA: Indomethacin [14, 15], Ibuprofen [16, 17], and surgical ligation [18] all are extremely effective in closing a PDA.

However, the focus of treatment should not be to close the PDA but to improve (long-term) outcome. And although the above-mentioned treatments for PDA effectively close the duct in the majority of patients, there is yet insufficient data on long-term consequences of such therapeutic interventions. An evidence-based approach to the treatment of PDA requires to weigh benefits and adverse effects of any therapy and to take the long-term consequences of treatment into consideration – particularly in our preterm patients who yet have all their life ahead.

Prophylactic Interventions

In the past, 28 randomized controlled trials enrolling 3965 preterm infants studied prophylactic interventions, both medical or surgical, aiming at closure of the ductus arteriosus [2].

Prophylactic ibuprofen, in contrast to prophylactic indomethacin, failed to reduce intraventricular hemorrhage [19], and prophylactic ligation was associated with an increased risk of chronic lung disease [20]. Both approaches do not seem to deserve further study at present.

The fundamental underlying questions for prophylactic use of indomethacin were:

- **P:** in preterm infants with less than 1000 g birth weight
- **I:** does prophylactic indomethacin (3 × 0.1 mg/kg q 24 h) started at ≤6 h
- **C:** compared with placebo
- **O:**
  - reduce PDA?
  - reduce intraventricular hemorrhage or periventricular hemorrhagic infarction?
  - reduce chronic lung disease of prematurity?
  - reduce death and neurodevelopmental impairment?

The answer to these questions is that although prophylactic indomethacin reduces the incidence of PDA requiring therapy and of severe intraventricular hemorrhage, it does not improve long-term neurodevelopment nor does it reduce the incidence of chronic lung disease [21]. These results have been confirmed in a recent meta-analysis [22].

The TIPP trial referenced above [21] was designed to prove a relative risk reduction of 25% (i.e., a difference in the incidence of death or NDI of 30% vs. 22.5% [Barbara Schmidt, personal communication]). The TIPP trial was not designed to prove that there is *no* difference in long-term outcome or to prove or exclude a smaller difference (either to the better or to the worse) in the incidence of death or NDI. Therefore, it is yet a matter of debate whether there may be a more subtle beneficial effect on neurodevelopmental outcome based on the reduction of severe intraventricular hemorrhage [23], although in the TIPP trial there was not even a trend towards an improved outcome.

The lack of a beneficial effect of prophylactic indomethacin on the incidence of chronic lung disease and neurodevelopmental impairment in the

TIPP trial lead to the conclusion that indomethacin may harm infants, i.e., increase the risk of chronic lung disease in patients in whom the PDA would have closed spontaneously [24], and may even impair neurodevelopment in infants not suffering from intraventricular hemorrhage. The TIPP investigators concluded that "indomethacin prophylaxis should not be prescribed with the expectation that the chances of survival without neurosensory impairment will be improved" [21] and others concluded that "a reduction of serious IVH with prophylactic use [of indomethacin] may justify this practice in selected high-risk patients, although the criteria are subject to debate" [25].

Consequently, the first pressing research question with regard to a prophylactic intervention is:

Q1: Is there a "high-risk" population in which a prophylactic intervention to close the duct results in long-term benefits?

Such a high-risk population would probably have to include the most immature infants, who are at particular risk of prolonged ductal patency and severe intraventricular hemorrhage. This population would have to include more boys than girls because boys are at a higher risk of an adverse outcome [26] and seem to benefit more from prophylactic indomethacin than girls [27]. The lack of spontaneous constriction of the duct during the first hours of life has been identified as a risk factor for later symptomatic PDA [6], pulmonary hemorrhage [6], and intraventricular hemorrhage [9] – as discussed in detail by Nick Evans in chapter 3. It is therefore probably also appropriate to focus prophylactic interventions on those infants with a widely open, non-constricted duct.

With respect to avoiding the potential adverse consequences of prophylactic administration of indomethacin outlined above, a reduction in the number of doses of indomethacin seems to be desireable, and such a reduction has been described before based on results of serial echocardiographic evaluations during treatment [28, 29]. Both studies, however, were too small to assess the risk/benefit ratio of such an approach and hence the second research question with regard to prophylactic intervention is:

Q2: Will a reduction in doses of indomethacin, e.g., guided by echocardiography, maintain its beneficial effects (reduction in the incidence of PDA and intraventricular hemorrhage) and reduce harmful effects of prophylactic indomethacin sufficiently to produce a net long-term benefit?

Both research questions, Q1 and Q2, could be addressed by a sufficiently powered study with the following design:

- ▬ **P:** in male infants <26 weeks and female infants <25 weeks, who do have a non-constricted duct at 4–6 h of life
- ▬ **I:** does prophylactic indomethacin (1–3 × 0,1 mg/kg q 24 h guided by echocardiography and started at ≤6 h)
- ▬ **C:** compared with placebo
- ▬ **O:** reduce neurodevelopmental impairment?

Therapeutic Interventions

Twenty randomized controlled trials have been performed to compare earlier with somewhat later interventions to close a persistently open duct. These trials enrolled only 796 preterm with no other apparent benefit than that the duct was closed earlier [2, 30–32].

Therapeutic trials performed to date have several limitations which will be addressed below.

The Problem of Indications for Treatment, i.e., the Definition of a PDA Requiring Therapy

Whereas prophylactic interventions have yet been applied to unselected patient populations who fulfilled some criteria related to prematurity, therapeutic interventions have to include patients based on the concept of a PDA requiring therapy. Such concepts have frequently used the term "hemodynamically significant PDA". Because it is yet impossible to reliably quantify the volume of a shunt through the open duct, definitions of a "hemodynamically significant PDA" are based on indirect indicators for a large shunt. These indicators have not been prospectively compared – probably because of a lack of an unequivocal gold standard, and it remains unclear which of these indicators most reliably indicates a PDA that impairs systemic and pulmonary hemodynamics to a degree that justifies treatment. We do not know whether e. g. a PDA with a diameter >1.5 mm, with reduced superior vena cava flow, with left atrial enlargement, a reduced LVPEP/LVET, an RI >0.9 in a peripheral artery or an increased BNP/cTNT indeed requires therapy.

These parametres are more extensively discussed by Eva Robel-Tillig in chapter 4 and Nick Evans in chapter 3.

Although all these parameters suggest some degree of alteration in hemodynamics compared with the circulatory situation of a closed duct, the relevance for patient outcome has not been proven for any. Similarly, the concept of staging a PDA according to clinical and echocardiographic characteristics [33] has not been evaluated prospectively with regard to patient outcome.

Instead of the concept of a "hemodynamically significant" PDA, the concept of a PDA "requiring therapy", defined as a PDA in which a therapeutic intervention to close it will improve outcome, should be introduced and supported by interventional trials. So far, the characteristics of a PDA requiring therapy according to this new definition are unknown. Consequently, the first and most important research question for therapeutic interventions for an open duct is:

Q1: Is there a PDA in which a therapeutic intervention to close it will improve outcome?

The Problem of Contamination

Most of the randomized controlled trials on therapeutic interventions aiming to close a PDA compared immediate with delayed treatment. Very few trials studied treatment versus placebo, and all of these offered later symptomatic treatment in up to 50% of patients in the control/placebo group. Contamination, however, reduces the measurable beneficial and harmful effects of the intervention investigated. Because in the end, all PDAs considered to be a problem were closed either by secondary medical interventions or surgical ligation, one cannot conclude that the lack of benefits with regard to the incidence of chronic lung disease or other complications of prematurity described in the meta-analyses mentioned above means that there is no benefit from therapy at all.

Any future study should therefore limit interventions to close a PDA in the control group. The second question for therapeutic interventions for an open duct is therefore:

Q2: Can we design a study in which contamination is negligible?

The Lack of Data on Long-Term Outcome

Although there are numerous trials there is no data on long-term outcome either for early pre-symptomatic treatment [32] nor for later symptomatic treatment [30, 31]. And the third most pressing question is consequently:

Q3: *Is there a therapeutic intervention for PDA that will result in improved medium- and long-term outcome?*
These research questions, **Q1** through **Q3**, could be addressed by a sufficiently powered study with the following design:

– **P:** In preterm infants <30 weeks with PDA meeting 4 of the following 5 criteria:
  – min. diameter >1.5 mm/kg,
  – pulsatile LR-Shunt ($v_{mindiast}$ <0.5 m/s),
  – negative or zero flow enddiastolic in the ACA,
  – negative or zero flow enddiastolic in the Coeliac Art.,
  – LA:Ao ratio >1.8, will
– **I:** does indomethacin (1–3 × 0.2–0.25 mg/kg i.v. q 12 h)
– **C:** compared with placebo "*and rescue only if intractable congestive heart failure develops*" (as suggested by Mathew Laughon [34])
– **O:** reduce death or neurodevelopmental impairment?

Further Open Questions

There are many open questions with respect to the treatment of PDA, however, these questions appear to be of lesser priority compared to those listed above and can be resolved once a population of preterm infants has been identified in whom treatment will result in improved outcome.

Which type of drug (i.e., indomethacin or ibuprofen) should be used?
Although a recent Cochrane review comes to the conclusion that ibuprofen is associated with less evidence of transient renal insufficiency (20 RCTs, 1092 pts) and a reduced incidence of necrotizing enterocolitis (15 RCTs, 865 infants) [35], particularly the later can only be considered a preliminary finding based on the marginal level of significance and the fact that 29 outcomes were evaluated in this review.

Do shortened courses (e.g., guided by echocardiography) improve outcome?
Two small studies reported a significant reduction in the number of doses required with an echocardiography-guided approach [28, 29]. However, apart from similar PDA closure rates, no effects on outcome were reported.

Do high dose courses improve outcome in case of persistent patency of the duct?
There is insufficient data to support the approach described by Sperandio and coworkers [36]. In particular, the trial was underpowered to detect less common complications such as intestinal perforation resulting from high-dose indomethacin.

Will continuous administration improve outcome compared to bolus administration?
There is insufficient data to draw any conclusion [37].

Do prolonged courses improve outcome?
The available data do not support the use of prolonged courses, but the trials were underpowered to detect small but relevant difference [38].

What is the preferred route of administration (i.e., i.v. versus i.m. verus oral)?
There is insufficient data to draw firm conclusion of data from the trials yet performed (e.g., [39]).

Which co-interventions will improve outcome in infants with an open duct?
Although there are pathophysiological arguments and very limited clinical data supporting that fluid restriction [40, 41], high levels of PEEP [41], permissive hypercapnia, and the use of dopamine [42, 43] and diuretics [44] may be associated with a reduction in pulmonary hyper- or systemic hypoperfusion, there is still insufficient data to make any final recommendations.

Summary

Unfortunately, we still do not know which PDA should be treated, i.e., we do not know what the echocardiographic, clinical, or biochemical characteristics of a PDA are, in which treatment will improve outcome.

We still do not know whether there is a high risk population that benefits from prophylactic intervention, and we still do not know which type/dose/length/route of treatment should be used and which additional therapies will support the infant best.

We also do not know whether we should ever ligate a PDA.

Thus, there remain plenty of studies to be performed to elucidate the optimal treatment for the patent arterial duct in preterm infants in the next 50 years to come.

References

1. Burnard ED (1959) The cardiac murmur in relation to symptoms in the newborn. Br Med J 1: 134–138
2. Benitz WE (2010) Treatment of persistent patent ductus arteriosus in preterm infants: time to accept the null hypothesis? J Perinatol 30: 241–252
3. Marshall DD, Kotelchuck M, Young TE et al. (1999) Risk factors for chronic lung disease in the surfactant era: a North Carolina population-based study of very low birth weight infants. North Carolina Neonatologists Association. Pediatrics 104: 1345–1350
4. Redline RW, Wilson-Costello D, Hack M (2002) Placental and other perinatal risk factors for chronic lung disease in very low birth weight infants. Pediatr Res 52: 713–719
5. Oh W, Poindexter BB, Perritt R et al. (2005) Association between fluid intake and weight loss during the first ten days of life and risk of bronchopulmonary dysplasia in extremely low birth weight infants. J Pediatr 147: 786–790
6. Kluckow M, Evans N (2000) Ductal shunting, high pulmonary blood flow, and pulmonary hemorrhage. J Pediatr 137: 68–72
7. Dollberg S, Lusky A, Reichman B (2005) Patent ductus arteriosus, indomethacin and necrotizing enterocolitis in very low birth weight infants: a population-based study. J Pediatr Gastroenterol Nutr 40: 184–188
8. Dykes FD, Lazzara A, Ahmann P et al. (1980) Intraventricular hemorrhage: a prospective evaluation of etiopathogenesis. Pediatrics 66: 42–49
9. Evans N, Kluckow M (1996) Early ductal shunting and intraventricular haemorrhage in ventilated preterm infants. Arch Dis Child Fetal Neonatal Ed 75: F183–186
10. Shortland DB, Gibson NA, Levene MI et al. (1990) Patent ductus arteriosus and cerebral circulation in preterm infants. Dev Med Child Neurol 32: 386–393
11. Drougia A, Giapros V, Krallis N et al. (2007) Incidence and risk factors for cerebral palsy in infants with perinatal problems: a 15-year review. Early Hum Dev 83: 541–547
12. Brooks JM, Travadi JN, Patole SK, Doherty DA, Simmer K (2005) Is surgical ligation of patent ductus arteriosus necessary? The Western Australian experience of conservative management. Arch Dis Child Fetal Neonatal Ed 90: F235–239
13. Noori S, McCoy M, Friedlich P et al. (2009) Failure of ductus arteriosus closure is associated with increased mortality in preterm infants. Pediatrics 123: e138–144

14. Friedman WF, Hirschklau MJ, Printz MP, Pitlick PT, Kirkpatrick SE (1976) Pharmacologic closure of patent ductus arteriosus in the premature infant. N Engl J Med 295: 526–529
15. Heymann MA, Rudolph AM, Silverman NH (1976) Closure of the ductus arteriosus in premature infants by inhibition of prostaglandin synthesis. N Engl J Med 295: 530–533
16. Patel J, Marks KA, Roberts I, Azzopardi D, Edwards AD (1995) Ibuprofen treatment of patent ductus arteriosus. Lancet 346: 255
17. Varvarigou A, Bardin CL, Beharry K et al. (1996) Early ibuprofen administration to prevent patent ductus arteriosus in premature newborn infants. JAMA 275: 539–544
18. Kitterman JA, Edmunds LH Jr, Gregory GA et al. (1972) Patent ducts arteriosus in premature infants. Incidence, relation to pulmonary disease and management. N Engl J Med 287: 473–477
19. Van Overmeire B, Allegaert K, Casaer A et al. (2004) Prophylactic ibuprofen in premature infants: a multicentre, randomised, double-blind, placebo-controlled trial. Lancet 364: 1945–1949
20. Clyman R, Cassady G, Kirklin JK, Collins M, Philips JB 3rd (2009) The role of patent ductus arteriosus ligation in bronchopulmonary dysplasia: reexamining a randomized controlled trial. J Pediatr 154: 873–876
21. Schmidt B, Davis P, Moddemann D et al. (2001) Long-term effects of indomethacin prophylaxis in extremely-low-birth-weight infants. N Engl J Med 344: 1966–1972
22. Fowlie PW, Davis PG, McGuire W (2010) Prophylactic intravenous indomethacin for preventing mortality and morbidity in preterm infants. Cochrane Database Syst Rev CD000174
23. Clyman RI, Saha S, Jobe A, Oh W (2007) Indomethacin prophylaxis for preterm infants: the impact of 2 multicentered randomized controlled trials on clinical practice. J Pediatr 150: 46–50 e2
24. Schmidt B, Roberts RS, Fanaroff A et al. (2006) Indomethacin prophylaxis, patent ductus arteriosus, and the risk of bronchopulmonary dysplasia: further analyses from the Trial of Indomethacin Prophylaxis in Preterms (TIPP). J Pediatr 148: 730–734
25. Hamrick SE, Hansmann G (2010) Patent ductus arteriosus of the preterm infant. Pediatrics 125: 1020–1030
26. Vohr BR, Allan WC, Westerveld M et al. (2003) School-age outcomes of very low birth weight infants in the indomethacin intraventricular hemorrhage prevention trial. Pediatrics 111: e340–346
27. Ment LR, Vohr BR, Makuch RW et al. (2004) Prevention of intraventricular hemorrhage by indomethacin in male preterm infants. J Pediatr 145: 832–834
28. Su BH, Peng CT, Tsai CH (1999) Echocardiographic flow pattern of patent ductus arteriosus: a guide to indomethacin treatment in premature infants. Arch Dis Child Fetal Neonatal Ed 81: F197–200
29. Carmo KB, Evans N, Paradisis M (2009) Duration of indomethacin treatment of the preterm patent ductus arteriosus as directed by echocardiography. J Pediatr 155: 819–822 e1
30. Clyman RI (1996) Recommendations for the postnatal use of indomethacin: an analysis of four separate treatment strategies. J Pediatr 128: 601–607
31. Knight DB (2001) The treatment of patent ductus arteriosus in preterm infants. A review and overview of randomized trials. Semin Neonatol 6: 63–73

32. Cooke L, Steer P, Woodgate P (2003) Indomethacin for asymptomatic patent ductus arteriosus in preterm infants. Cochrane Database Syst Rev CD003745

33. McNamara PJ, Sehgal A (2007) Towards rational management of the patent ductus arteriosus: the need for disease staging. Arch Dis Child Fetal Neonatal Ed 92: F424–427

34. Laughon MM, Simmons MA, Bose CL (2004) Patency of the ductus arteriosus in the premature infant: is it pathologic? Should it be treated? Curr Opin Pediatr 16: 146–151

35. Ohlsson A, Walia R, Shah SS (2010) Ibuprofen for the treatment of patent ductus arteriosus in preterm and/or low birth weight infants. Cochrane Database Syst Rev: CD003481

36. Sperandio M, Beedgen B, Feneberg R et al. (2005) Effectiveness and side effects of an escalating, stepwise approach to indomethacin treatment for symptomatic patent ductus arteriosus in premature infants below 33 weeks of gestation. Pediatrics 116: 1361–1366

37. Gork AS, Ehrenkranz RA, Bracken MB (2008) Continuous infusion versus intermittent bolus doses of indomethacin for patent ductus arteriosus closure in symptomatic preterm infants. Cochrane Database Syst Rev: CD006071

38. Herrera C, Holberton J, Davis P (2007) Prolonged versus short course of indomethacin for the treatment of patent ductus arteriosus in preterm infants. Cochrane Database Syst Rev: CD003480

39. Aly H, Lotfy W, Badrawi N et al. (2007) Oral Ibuprofen and ductus arteriosus in premature infants: a randomized pilot study. Am J Perinatol 24: 267–270

40. Bell EF, Acarregui MJ (2008) Restricted versus liberal water intake for preventing morbidity and mortality in preterm infants. Cochrane Database Syst Rev: CD000503

41. Vanhaesebrouck S, Zonnenberg I, Vandervoort P et al. (2007) Conservative treatment for patent ductus arteriosus in the preterm. Arch Dis Child Fetal Neonatal Ed 92: F244–247

42. Barrington K, Brion LP (2002) Dopamine versus no treatment to prevent renal dysfunction in indomethacin-treated preterm newborn infants. Cochrane Database Syst Rev: CD003213

43. Bouissou A, Rakza T, Klosowski S et al. (2008) Hypotension in preterm infants with significant patent ductus arteriosus: effects of dopamine. J Pediatr 153: 790–794

44. Brion LP, Campbell DE (2001) Furosemide for symptomatic patent ductus arteriosus in indomethacin-treated infants. Cochrane Database Syst Rev: CD001148

Summary of the Discussions During the International Workshop on "Controversies Around Treatment of the Patent Ductus Arteriosus"

P. Herrmann

This report summarizes the discussions held in Stuttgart during a two-day workshop (September 30 to October 1, 2010, in Stuttgart, Germany) on "Controversies around Treatment of the Patent Ductus Arteriosus" sponsored by Orphan Europe. The aim of the meeting was to discuss the different approaches taken in the management of PDA. Internationally-renowned speakers and attending participants exchanged experiences and views about when and whether to treat or not to treat patent ductus arteriosus (PDA), which rationale to follow in selecting appropriate treatment, and how the results of various studies on different drugs and dosages are shaping the guidelines for the future management of PDA. The focus was also directed to other important aspects relating to this group of patients, such as the role of echocardiography and Doppler imaging.

In the first lecture on "Ductal Closure After Birth", delivered by **Regina Bökenkamp** (Leiden, The Netherlands), it was pointed out that ductal closure after birth occurs via contraction and anatomical remodelling; with the contraction of smooth muscle cells being attended by an increase in PO_2 and withdrawal of prostaglandin (PG). During anatomical remodelling, which starts during the second trimester of pregnancy, intima cushions are formed via prostaglandin signalling. In replying to the first question raised by participants, about whether attempts had been made to alter these cushions pharmacologically, Dr. Bökenkamp explained that gene transfer methods had been used to block the formation of cushions in lambs. The focus of the remaining queries was on treatment and Dr. Bökenkamp clarified that, in an Australian study done 10 years ago, the effect of synthetic PG was similar to PG1, with the dosage starting at 0.05 mcg/kg/min and decreasing to a maintenance dose of 0.01 mcg/kg/min. However, participants pointed out that, in the Netherlands, for instance, the general treatment trend over the last two years was to start with lower doses immediately after birth.

After the first speaker, **Petra Koehne** (Berlin, Germany), presented the "Treatment Results After Ductal Closure in Extremely Low Gestational Age Infants", several questions were raised about the three lines of treatment currently applied: ibuprofen treatment, indomethacin therapy and surgical ligation. Dr. Koehne described the neurodevelopmental outcome, at two years' corrected age, of VLBW infants who were treated with indomethacin (n=89) or ibuprofen (n=93) for a hemodynamically significant PDA at her hospital between 1998 and 2003. She also highlighted the two-year outcome results for the subgroup of infants (n=54) in whom COX inhibitor treatment failed, and who subsequently underwent PDA ligation. In assessing the early outcome of surgical ligation, Dr. Koehne presented the results of her group which showed that serious side-effects had been observed after ligation, such as tension pneumothorax, pneumoperitoneum, intraoperative bleeding, pulmonary hemorrhage, phrenic palsy and wound infection. Participants also drew attention to nerve findings, by referring to a study, in Denmark, by Gorm Greisen and colleagues, in which a total mortality of 15% was found among babies who had undergone surgical ligation within a period of four months.

The discussion focused on whether ligation should only be done when treatment with ibuprofen or indomethacin failed to achieve ductal closure. Dr. Koehne explained that, at her hospital, ligation is only carried out in infants who are still being mechanically ventilated and when extubation was not feasible. She pointed out that her unit was fortunate to have a cardiac surgeon from the German Heart Institute at hand, which made it possible for the procedure to be carried out in the NICU itself. She remarked that the risk associated with transportation led to a bias in some studies and that this risk was avoidable due to the favourable circumstances in her center.

Dr. Koehne cautioned against taking a hasty decision to introduce prophylatic medication when abdominal distension or early stages of NEC were observed. In her unit, a "wait and see" approach was taken as these signs were considered contraindications for treatment.

In fielding questions about the line of treatment to follow when ibuprofen failed, she emphasized that such a decision could only be made by considering each case on an individual basis. She recommended prolonging the medication and considering a higher dose, as studies had shown that drug metabolism via cytochrome P450 enzymes possibly increases as the child's age progresses. Studies of low numbers of patients under such regimes provide limited knowledge. In her experience, a second cycle did not always prove to be beneficial. She regarded the child's post-natal age and ductal diameter as important aspects to consider before scheduling a second cycle.

Dr. Koehne remarked that, in a recent network meta-analysis, ibuprofen was associated with an approximately 30% greater risk of chronic lung disease (CLD) in comparison to indomethacin. In the meta-analysis, bronchopulmonary dysplasia (BPD) was evident on day 28; however, Thomas et al. did not observe this at a corrected age of 36 weeks.

In his lecture on "Echocardiographic Assessment of the Patent Ductus Arteriousus in the Preterm Infant", **Nick Evans** (Sydney, Australia) described how this imaging method was a reliable means of establishing an accurate diagnosis of PDA *before* clinical signs appear. He illustrated how early post-natal constriction predicts spontaneous closure and, in addition, how an early post-therapy constrictive response also predicts therapeutic closure. The hemodynamic impact is often evident at an early stage in babies with significant ducts. The dilemma of when to treat a PDA, however, remained unresolved due to the wide range of differences in early ductal constriction, the implications of early shunting, subsequent post-natal constriction as well as response to treatment.

He clarified that, instead of analyzing Doppler velocities of peripheral, cerebral or mesenteric arteries, it would probably be more relevant to focus on the blood-flow patterns through and near the duct. He stated that the primary focus should be on the ductal size and shunt pattern but that diastolic flow patterns in the descending aorta and left pulmonary artery were useful ancillary measures. It was important to remember that Doppler measurements of peripheral arteries were markers of flow pattern rather than of the flow volume. He explained that absent or reverse diastolic flow was not necessarily evidence of low flow and that the status of diastolic flow velocity may not be particularly important if good systolic flow was observable.

Participants pointed out that, since there was wide variation in the rate of ductal closure of preterms, the six-hour cut-off would be appropriate in babies with quick constriction, but not for cases in which the constriction process is slower. It was argued that slower constriction was not necessarily pathological and that it might be more appropriate to extend the cut-off to 24 hours or even further to 72 hours. Dr. Evans clarified that, at the moment, treatment in his hospital is being directed by a clinical trial of very early, echo-targeted treatment compared to later treatment directed by the development of signs or symptoms of ductal shunting. Both groups had the option of rescue treatment if necessary.

In replying to a comment about the lack of evidence of the benefit of bedside echocardiography and how the time utilized for it would lead to less time for other procedures, Dr. Evans emphasized that this was a diagnostic modality and that almost none of the many diagnostic modalities used in neonatology were supported by clinical trial evidence showing benefit. Accuracy was important to test, however, in terms of evidence development it was crucial to consider what is done with the information. While often criticised for its potential to lead to over-intervention, experimental clinician-performed ultrasound was just as likely to give the treating physician the confidence *not* to intervene. He recounted several instances of babies in his hospital who would not have survived if an echocardiogram had not been performed in a timely manner.

In her lecture on the "Evaluation of the Open Duct Using Systolic Time Intervals and Doppler Sonography of Peripheral Arteries", **Eva Robel-Tillig** (Leipzig, Germany) highlighted the need to measure parameters of two or three vessels. Significant PDA in neonates was strongly associated with disturbances in organ blood flow, and several measurements of blood-flow velocity and pulsatility index had proven valuable in assessing the cardiocirculatory effects of PDA. These included the blood flow of the descending aorta and the celiac access as well as the flow in cerebral, mesenteric and renal blood vessels. Additionally, Doppler flow parameters of cerebral, renal or mesenteric arteries provided valuable information about whether PDA in a given preterm is hemodynamic or not. Measurements of systolic time intervals were not only valuable, but also represented a quick, non-invasive method that was easy to learn, with the added advantage that it involved low stress levels in neonates.

The discussion focused on the practical aspects relating to treatment. Dr. Robel-Tillig underscored the fact that, in the study she presented, the decision to treat a neonate was based on typical findings, such as high left ventricular cardiac output, disturbed time intervals or disturbances in organ blood flow parameters in two peripheral vessels. She remarked that the predictive value of disturbed diastolic flow in two vessels had a high specificity and that ultrasound of the duct was still the "gold standard" in making a decision about not to treat. In ducts that continue to be open after treatment, it would be useful to study the time intervals, since depressed myocardial function is accompanied by prolongation of the left ventricular pre-ejection period (LPEP).

Luc Desfrère (Paris, France) delivered a lecture on the "Competitive Inhibition of Bilirubin-Albumin Binding by Ibuprofen", in which he described the results of a study conducted at his hospital, from 2004 to 2007, on the safety of ibuprofen in treating hyperbilirubinemic preterms with PDA. He explained that drugs such as ibuprofen could lead to the displacement of bilirubin from albumin binding, and, as a result, an increase in unbound bilirubin (UB) could occur, which, in turn, could lead to neurotoxicity. The displacing effect had been observed in vitro when high amounts (>100–200 mcg/mL) of ibuprofen were applied. He remarked that although UB was considered a critical parameter in assessing bilirubin toxicity, the issue relating to the interaction between bilirubin, albumin and ibuprofen had yet to be resolved. Participants were eager to know whether the study results could confirm that phototherapy influenced the metabolism of UB and thereby reduced its toxicity. Dr. Desfrère stated that all the patients in his study had undergone phototherapy; however, the screening for bilirubin toxicity did not involve examining the influence of this treatment.

Participants pointed out that, since the sample size was small (n=34), the conclusion that ibuprofen treatment was probably safe, needs to be confirmed in a larger trial. There was general consensus about in vitro and ex vivo studies being important steps in gaining more insight into this question. Randomized trials were crucial for studying the interaction between blood components and different drugs. It was suggested that, since Dr. Desfrère's study showed that ibuprofen was marginally better than indomethacin, the time had probably come to do the right trial.

The second day began with a session titled "Prophylactic Versus Late Treatment of PDA – a Pro-Con Debate", with **Bart Van Overmeire** (Brussels, Belgium) taking the "pro" standpoint and **Barbara Schmidt** (Philadelphia, USA) representing the "con" point of view.

The first question posed by participants was whether it was acceptable to interpret tendencies or data that were clearly insignificant. Dr. Schmidt's emphatic response was that it was important to look at trends, provided adequate caution was taken, particularly at the bedside. She explained that a critical look at trends is not to be equated with endorsing or even proving a given therapy, which is why her studies have at no time claimed that prophylactic indomethacin is per se harmful or causes 'the better babies' to do worse. She argued that statistics from studies were sometimes merely "a trade-off of numbers": She referred to the TIPP study in which some babies did worse than others in a given sub-group, and at 18 months the number of cases with severe intraventricular hemorrhage (IVH) reduced by one-third. She stressed how important it was for junior physicians to depart from the well-trodden path of thinking, in which a p-value of 0.049 was proof that a substance was beneficial but a p-value of 0.051 was proof of its ineffectiveness.

Questions to the "pro" standpoint focused on blood vessels. Participants from Germany confirmed that the decrease in diastolic flow referred to by Dr. Van Overmeire, was a finding generally evident in ultrasound scans. It was reported that, in children with PDA, the function of vessel density decreased; however, the distribution of vessels changed: a decrease of larger vessels was observed in the microcirculation of larger vessels and, concurrently, a significant increase in the various small capillaries, last-stage vessels occurred. It was thought that the delivery of oxygen and nutrients to tissue remained unaffected due to the counteracting forces associated with an increase of smaller vessels, as these were the "final gatekeepers" of how much is ultimately conveyed. This was similar to the Doppler effect on very large vessels, in which large vessels were known to produce the greatest part of the signal.

Dr. Van Overmeire clarified that, on the microscopic level, some babies with PDA could compensate for the negative effects, depending on the type of PDA and the direction of the shunt. However, he thought that, at a certain level, the flow and the impact of the PDA would be rather strong and, as a result, compensatory mechanisms would probably fail. Thus, it may not be able to compensate for the high impact of a large PDA. He said the physician was now confronted by two questions: firstly, which PDA or shunt is large enough to merit treatment and secondly, when is it appropriate to wait and see because the baby was doing well, while presuming, at the microcirculatory level, that this approach probably did no harm.

Dr. Van Overmeire asked the participants whether they would find it useful to have a device at the bedside, in future, to assess the situation in the brain or in the body at that level. The replies indicated that some participants had successfully done this without knowing which child had a PDA and found it was a cumbersome process, adding that studies had yet to be done. It was now technically possible to look at the oxygen content of these very small vessels by means of a microcirculatory video. Because this was an external method, however, the brain could not be examined and it might be more useful to have biochemical markers, one candidate possibly being troponin.

Participants were very appreciative about the compelling physiological evidence presented by Dr. Van Overmeire, which showed that PDA does provide a potential insult. Participants expanded on this view by stating that the nature of all human injury is such that every individual responds differently to the same insult. It was generally – wrongly – assumed that an insult had a homogeneous effect in a group of individuals.

Participants stated that this also applied to the context of randomized trials and systematic reviews: The assumption prevailed that the benefits and harms of the PDA effect are evenly distributed across the population. It was pointed out that Dr. Schmidt had shown that there may actually be a group of babies who benefited and, on the other hand, a group which would be harmed. It was necessary to look more closely in order to identify the babies who would benefit and distinguish them from the others.

Interesting parallels were found with regard to post-natal steroids: data of their harm dominated in studies in which all babies received significant doses from early on, with the drug thus maximizing the harm. Dr. Schmidt agreed with this view and pointed out that, although this was a debate, the "pro" and "con" positions were not very far from each other. She clarified that while physiology did matter, it did not suffice on its own. Those who work out a principle on a physiological basis must test it with real patients and also test for clinically important outcomes.

She reminded participants that the host of well-designed, enormously successful randomized trials in adult cardiology had started out as small trials which examined surrogate outcomes that included physiological outcomes. She recalled that when a new class of promising anti-arrhythmic drugs were introduced, they were very effective, in terms of returning arrhythmias to the sinus rhythm. It was prescribed to thousands of people and, ultimately, proved fatal. It had been estimated that more people in the USA died due to this drug than in the Vietnam War. She said that this was a very powerful reminder of how one should not stop with physiology data but that both were needed.

A participant from Austria said his hospital took a prophylactic approach: at the end of day 1, when the baby had good diuresis, a very low dose of indomethacin (0.05 mg per dose) was given. No ligations had been done in the last 10 years, one reason being the IVH prophylaxis, which, however, had not been tested in a randomized controlled study. He wanted to know whether any studies comparing dosages had been done, for instance in a prophylactic trial with a very low dose having a good effect but causing less side-effects.

Dr. Van Overmeire described a recent paper that did not involve a prophylaxis but which compared the standard dose of indomethacin in 24-hour intervals during the first week of life, with a dosage of about 0.2 or 0.1 mg of indomethacin. A 12-hour interval was applied in the second group, which showed a higher efficacy and a similar rate of side-effects. Studies of ibuprofen as well as indomethacin showed high variability in pharmacokinetics and pharmacodynamics in these babies, and that the volume of distribution was different in all cases, i.e., some were hypervolemic, others hypovolemic. Generally, lower doses were given to younger babies, and the dose was increased as age advanced in order to achieve the same effect.

Dr. Schmidt added that the TIPP trial set the dose at 0.1 mg/kg every 24 h, starting soon after birth, mainly because the babies had to be recruited within six hours of birth. The reasoning was that an early start was needed to find out whether one of the effects occurs through preventing IVH. The lowest bracket of dosage was chosen from studies that had shown their effectiveness on short-term outcomes.

Dr. Van Overmeire further clarified that the speed of the indomethacin injection also had an effect and if it was given in a fast bolus, it had additional vasoconstrictive effects on the brain. He thought that a prophylaxis, given in a continuous or a low dose, as in Austria, may be quite different from a higher dose given as a bolus. To his knowledge, such an interesting trial had not been done on a large scale.

He raised the question about which criterion was appropriate for ligation. In his experience, different approaches were taken: in some units it was common to prescribe pharmacological treatment and, if the patent duct was still there and the baby was on CPAP or still needed oxygen, he called for the surgeon.

Fewer ligations were a positive development and he raised the question about whether some centers opt for ligation too hastily. Dr. Schmidt agreed with this point and mentioned that this issue was the objective of a study that Kishore Kabra had published with her group. She stated that the variability in the ligation rate in the international centers was remarkable and that, in the unadjusted analysis, they saw an effect which showed that the centers with the lowest rate had the best long-term outcomes. When they adjusted it for baseline risk factors, the same "trend" remained but the conventional p-value cutpoint was lost, suggesting that differences in patient populations were related to these differences.

Dr. Evans stated that, when studying IVH serially, a group will be seen which includes about one-third of the patients, in whose cases IVH is present in the very early hours after birth. He argued that it would be logical to think that it was impossible to prevent something that had already taken place. On these grounds, he felt that Dr. Schmidt's criticism of the Laura Ment trial was unfounded. He said one of the problems related to the analyses of IVH was the fact that the babies were scanned on day 4 to day 7 and all the data were put together. He was aware that this was not included in the TIPP trial for pragmatic reasons; however, his view was that the design of the Laura Ment trial was more logical as they excluded those cases in whom what they were trying to prevent had already happened. Dr. Schmidt and Dr. Evans reached a consensus by describing the Laura Ment trial as a "mechanistically logical trial". Dr. Schmidt said her criticism was only directed at the fact that very few events were observed in that trial, and that, if the study would have the same design and would screen out the bad bleeds at the beginning, they would have needed 10 or 20 times the sample size! She acknowledged it was a trial studying the prevention of IVH with very few events. Both agreed that a bigger sub-group was needed in the Ment trial.

Dr. Christian Poets (Tuebingen, Germany) mentioned that his group found that, in the subgroup of infants with a GA of 24–25 weeks, 90% had been routinely treated with indomethacin in his institution. They reasoned that, by using indomethacin prophylactically in this subgroup of very immature infants, and by applying it only in a neonatal trial dose of 0.1 mg/kg, they would avoid unnecessary exposure to a therapeutic dose of indomethacin and thus expose only a very small fraction of infants to the higher dose.

Dr. Van Overmeire commented that today this might be a reasonable approach for a prophylaxis. In view of the discussion, he felt that it was possibly true that not every baby reacted in the same way, and that the benefit-risk ratio also varied. The studies mentioned, which showed differences between boys and girls, led him to suggest coming to a consensus about a prophylaxis for boys but not for girls – and thus partly closing the gap with the "con" standpoint.

Dr. Schmidt reiterated that sub-group analysis could never be used as a basis for treatment. She commended Dr. Poets' approach because he first considered his own data and combined that with published evidence before drawing conclusions relevant to his setting instead of "importing" published data without being able to investigate its viability on the local scene. She felt it sounded reasonable that 90% of these babies were exposed to indomethacin and presumed that the next speaker, Dr. Laughon, would probably challenge an approach in which 90% of the babies would be treated for a PDA.

Another participant referred to a slide shown by Dr. Van Overmeire, which showed that a duct that was patent for more than 7 days increased the risk of BPD. He pointed out that many of these studies did not make adjustments for risk factors that were also known to contribute to the development of BPD. For instance, his group had observed that the most immature preterms were those who were diagnosed with BPD. These infants also had serious infections, among other things. He felt it was important to be guided by the well-designed analyses and that small studies should only be considered if their analyses showed data adjusted for risks.

Dr. Van Overmeire said that this comment was a very important one, since it was commonly known that the problem was a multi-factorial one. Risk factors needed to be combined and this was a difficult task. For instance, if one wanted to reassess a study in order to check the rate of inflammation, the data did not necessarily have to include a proven infection established via positive microbial cultures. He thought that inflammation also played an important role.

The final point was brought up by Dr. Schmidt in order to clarify the question about the duration of PDA that kept coming up in the discussion. She emphasized that every physician had been confronted with the long-standing dogma that declared that: the longer the PDA persists, the worse it is. She referred to a figure in the paper she cited earlier (with co-author Kabra) on the possible risks of ligation. In that paper, they had plotted age at PDA ligation against the TIPP primary outcome of death or disability at 18 months. In keeping with that dogma, they hypothesized that earlier ligation would result in better outcomes; however, they did not find the trend of time they expected; in fact, hardly any type of effect was found.

The lecture by **Bernd Beedgen** (Heidelberg, Germany), on "High-Dose Therapy with Cyclooxygenase-Inhibitors for Symptomatic Persistent Ductus Arteriosus in Preterms" focused not only on his extended experience with indomethacin but also on new data on ibuprofen provided by his colleague Michael Schroth (Erlangen, Germany). Dr. Beedgen pointed out that although indomethacin was introduced 35 years ago, its risks and benefits are still being debated. He outlined a rather recent (2008) randomized study in the USA, which came to the conclusion that high-dose indomethacin could not be recommended at the time as it did not lead to significantly higher rates of PDA closure and was associated with an increased risk of moderate to severe retinopathy of prematurity (ROP). The study conducted by his own group, from 1993 to 2002, on the other hand, concluded that high-dose indomethacin at up to 1.0 mg/kg was an effective, safe treatment for symptomatic PDA.

Dr. Beedgen summarized the results of the successful high-dose regime with indomethecin by pointing out the higher closure rate of PDA and a lower rate of surgical ligation.

The discussion mainly focused on details of the indomethacin therapy. Participants asked whether the elimination rate of indomethacin differed among the studied babies; however, this was not measured in Dr. Beedgen's study.

In another German center, high-dose indomethacin was associated with a high rate of intestinal perforation, which led to the therapy being abandoned after six months. A decision against publication was made as the number of patients was very small; however, other participants felt it might be useful to have a published report of these findings.

Dr. Beedgen was cautious about offering recommendations on how to augment the dose; however, some participants suggested birth weight or current weight as guiding parameters.

"The Open Duct: Wait and See?" was the provocative title of the lecture delivered by **Matthew M. Laughon** (Chapel Hill, USA) in which he described the various controversies related to the management of PDA. After analyzing the factors influencing the decision of whether or how to treat, such as the rate of spontaneous closure, the risks associated with persistent patency, and the benefits and risks of treatments for closure, Dr. Laughon remarked that the strength of evidence ranged from systematic reviews and meta-analysis to single randomized controlled studies, single observational studies, physiologic studies and even unsystematic clinical observations. He argued that most studies were designed to test the efficacy of therapy and not the impact of persistent patency of the duct or the benefit of closure. He stated that all the studies permitted "back-up" treatment of the PDA with no true placebo group. Dr. Laughon concluded that such features of study design made it impossible to quantify the benefits and risks of therapies to close the PDA.

The question was therefore: What should the clinician do when the benefits and risks of a treatment are unknown? He described three types of clinicians: (1) The Empiricists, who base treatment on biological plausibility, anecdote or personal experience; (2) The Pragmatists, who decide to treat on the basis of the clinical evidence of benefit; and (3) The Nihilists, who only treat an infant if incontrovertible evidence shows that the benefits of therapy are greater than the risks. Finally, he argued that treatment modalities therefore depended on whether PDA was associated with CLD and necrotizing enterocolitis (NEC) and also on which categories of clinicians were involved in decisions on therapy.

Participants asked for Dr. Laughon's advice on when to perform surgical ligation or, instead, opt for high-dose treatment. He explained that his group had a lot of experience with ligations but not with high-dose treatment. They observed five groups of patients with ligation and found that those who were ligated were smaller than the babies receiving indomethacin. The short-term outcomes in the babies given indomethacin was deplorable (13% to 16% developing NEC) and probably represented a sicker group. He remarked that it was interesting to read a report from Australia which mentioned that one of the hospitals did not have a surgeon and the closest one was 1,000 miles away! He said it was understandable that this hospital did not carry out ligations for several years. It was even more interesting to note that there was no significant difference between groups in the incidence of CLD, CLD or death, necrotising enterocolitis, intraventricular hemorrhage, duration of oxygen, or hospital stay. He compared this to the rate of ligation in the TIPP trial, which ranged from 0% to 20%. Whereas in the past there were 300 to 400 ligations done in this trial, a turn around occurred in 2008, after which only one ligation had been performed.

In replying to a question about ligation and short-term mechanistic evidence relating to the hemodynamic effects of a PDA, Dr. Laughon referred to the efforts of the group working with Dr. Patrick McNamara in Toronto (Canada), which is preparing a staging system to characterize the clinical and echocardiographic impact of the ductus arteriosus. Comprehensive echocardiography evaluation will be used to assess ductal size and the degree of pulmonary overcirculation/systemic hypoperfusion related to the transductal shunt. Dr. Laughon pointed out that the staging system had still to be validated.

Participants remarked that it was frustrating to separate the non-treatment group from the treatment group, mainly because this was confounded by the investigators' biases. It was pointed out that the National Institute for Child Health and Human Development (NICHD) research network in the USA had set up a risk categorization initiative comprising two approaches: "do nothing" and "be pro-active".

"Missing Data for an Evidence-Based Approach to the Treatment of PDA" was the final lecture of the workshop, which **Axel Franz** (Tübingen, Germany) delivered.

Participants were keen to know whether, in Dr. Franz's unit, all babies under 30 weeks of gestation were given prophylactic treatment, and were informed that this was not at all the case. Dr. Franz explained that the focus was on the very premature babies and the current practice in the unit was to give a prophylaxis only to those infants with a predominant left-to-right shunt;

additionally, in infants less than 26 weeks of gestation, there should be no signs of duct-dependent circulation. He stated that, in a further step, one could probably limit treatment to female infants with a gestational age (GA) of less than 25 weeks and males with a GA of less than 26 weeks, provided the duct was larger than 1.5 mm in diameter.

Questions on the eligibility criteria for the trial being planned by Dr. Franz pertained to the intention to use prophylactic indomethacin in infants with a PDA larger than 1.5 mm at entry. It was argued that this criterion involved the implicit assumption that the prevention of IVH can be achieved via treatment for PDA, thus using an approach for which limited knowledge was available. Dr. Franz cited the circumstantial evidence collected by Dr. Evans' group, which showed that a large PDA was associated with lower flow in the superior vena cava – which, in turn, is associated with late IVH.

Dr. Evans and colleagues had done an analysis in order to determine whether the size of the duct needed to be corrected for weight. Their findings showed that weight was not an important determinant of size. In the 500–600 echocardiograms examined by this group, the predictive power was in the first 12 hours of life. The predominant determinant of the size of the duct was, in fact, not the size of the baby but the postnatal age, which is why Dr. Evans felt the new study might not need to correct ductal diameter for birthweight. He stated that his unit had a sliding scale which shows the medians of different post-natal ages. He suggested that it would be advantageous if the design of Dr. Franz's intended study would be as close to his as possible in order to facilitate good comparisons.

Dr. Franz explained that another reason for correcting the ductal diameter for weight was that smaller infants were more likely to have hemorrhage. He stated he would be willing to include smaller infants in the future study, and was rather reluctant to include the larger infants. He added, that correcting for birth weight would reduce the number of larger infants who met the inclusion criteria.

The very intention to include duct diameter in the entry criteria of the study was also questioned. It was argued that, during the process of selecting entry criteria, it was crucial to ensure that valid measurements could be made in a multi-center trial, otherwise a trial would conclude with a great deal of data which lacked coherence.

Subject Index

V

vascular smooth muscle cells (VSMCs) 7
ventriculomegaly 15
Vermont Oxford Network 126
very low birth weight (VLBW) infants 12, 82
Vineland Adaptive Behaviour Scales (VABS)
    102
– composite score 105
– subscale scores 105
vocal cord paralysis 116, 124

W

water restriction 82
white matter disease 87
wound infection 145

Printing: Ten Brink, Meppel, The Netherlands
Binding: Stürtz, Würzburg, Germany